AIRWAY DEVELOPMENT 101

A BEGINNER'S GUIDE TO IMPROVING BREATHING, SLEEP QUALITY, AND ORAL HEALTH FOR YOU AND YOUR CHILDREN WITHOUT COMPLICATED TECHNIQUES

DR. MARKUS WILSON DMD, BA

A special thanks to my sister, Lacey, whose professional insights and creative input have greatly influenced the content of this book. Your suggestions, patience, and enthusiasm have been invaluable.

TABLE OF CONTENTS

Introduction   7

1. THE TALE YOUR FACE TELLS   13
   Faces of the Past   13
   A Map of Breath and Life   18
   Why Airway Anatomy Matters   23
   Quick Recap   27

2. TAKE A DEEP BREATH   29
   The Art and Science of Breathing   29
   When Form Meets Function   34
   Breathing Trouble: Signs to Watch in Children   39
   Quick Recap   45

3. GROWING UP WITH A HEALTHY SMILE   47
   Foundations of a Healthy Face   48
   Curbing Detrimental Habits Early   54
   The Brain-Bite Connection   61
   It Is Time for Facial Fitness!   65
   Quick Recap   66

4. BREATHING RIGHT   69
   The Power of Proper Breathing   69
   Nasal Matters   72
   Why the Long Face?   75
   BreatheEasy 360 Method   77
   Breathing Exercises for the Little Ones   79
   Breathwork for School-Age Kids and Teens   82
   Quick Recap   86

5. LIFESTYLE CHOICES THAT COUNT   91
   Posture and Breathing   91
   Stand Tall   93
   Get Moving   96
   Quick Recap   103

6. CHEW ON THIS   105
    You Are What You Eat   105
    Essential Nutrients for a Winning Smile   111
    Crunch Time   120
    Quick Recap   123

7. SWEET DREAMS ARE MADE OF THESE   125
    The Breath of Night   126
    Recognizing Sleep Issues   129
    A Dreamy Sleep Environment   135
    Quick Recap   142

8. STRAIGHT TALK   145
    Orthodontics: Beyond a Beautiful Smile   146
    A Closer Look at Orthodontic Appliances   148
    Case Studies   152
    Timing Is Everything   154
    Quick Recap   158

9. A GOOD EXAMPLE   161
    Leading Your Brood   161
    Breathwork for Parents: Enhancing Your Own
    Health   165
    Posture for Parents   167
    Quick Recap   179

    Conclusion   183
    References   187

INTRODUCTION

As a child, I was troubled by a set of symptoms that seemed to defy explanation—large tonsils, crowded teeth, incessant snoring, poor sleep, and ever-present fatigue that clung to me like a relentless shadow. I never understood why my sleep was never as restful as that of my friends. I would wake up feeling more tired than when I went to bed, and I was always fatigued during the day. Little did I know that these seemingly different conditions were all linked to undiagnosed airway problems.

I became used to the noise of my own snoring—a dissonant lullaby that echoed through the night. My parents, too, grew accustomed to the restless sleep and the bags under my eyes that spoke volumes about the quality of my rest. At the time, the idea that these symptoms were a sign of a more serious health issue was a notion that eluded us.

During that time, my parents took me to several doctors seeking answers to the mysterious condition that troubled my every waking moment. The journey through the medical system was also full of challenges. Ear, nose, and throat (ENT) specialists—initially dismissive of the severity of my condition—hesitated to remove my enlarged tonsils, which left my parents and me frustrated. We felt trapped in a system that seemed indifferent to our struggles. Meanwhile, we booked several medical appointments but found conflicting opinions and moments of desperation that only made us more determined to find a solution.

My parents had to go through the whole healthcare system just yearning to end my suffering. They faced a lot of challenges—from systemic barriers to the reluctance of healthcare professionals to try out alternative treatments. Despite the notable toll this struggle took on our family, my parents' dedication inspired my resilience.

Despite the setbacks, I refused to give up. With determination and effort, I became my own advocate tirelessly navigating the healthcare system in search of answers. The journey was fraught with obstacles, but I refused to let them defeat me. Just when I was on the verge of giving up hope, a glimmer of light appeared on the horizon—a turning point that would change everything.

As I share this personal experience, I cannot help but acknowledge the countless parents who find themselves struggling with similar challenges. As parents, we have to encounter several challenges in this journey. The overwhelming responsibility we have seems to be huge. The fear of not meeting our children's needs adequately constantly haunts us. This anxiety comes from concerns about providing optimal care, support, and decision-making to ensure our children's growth. We question ourselves fearing that we might overlook vital information, fail to be proactive in addressing potential health issues, or make decisions that could impact our children's future health, happiness, and success.

Surrounding this emotional strain is the tangible distress caused by our children's breathing difficulties evident through symptoms like snoring, mouth breathing, or sleep apnea. These issues disrupt their sleep, which increases fatigue and the risk of more health problems. As parents, we also tend to struggle to find accessible and reliable information on how to improve our children's breathing, sleep quality, and oral health. The lack of comprehensive guidance further impedes making informed decisions and taking timely action, and this potentially results in delayed intervention and the worsening of existing problems. Also, our children's dental issues such as misaligned teeth, jaw disorders, or cavities add another layer of concern affecting not only oral health but also overall well-being and self-esteem—the most difficult challenges and experiences anyone should endure.

Yearning for a solution amid these challenges? Are you tired of feeling helpless whenever you see your child struggling with breathing? Do you find yourself questioning if you are doing enough to ensure their future health and happiness? Are you overwhelmed by the lack of accessible information? This is where this book comes into play.

Through this book, you will be introduced to the BreatheEasy 360 method—a holistic approach to improving your child's airway health. From sleep patterns to facial development, lifestyle, and environment, this method covers all the bases and provides you with practical, everyday steps that you can take to make a real difference in your child's respiratory health.

So, what is the end result? This book promises a life where your child sleeps soundly, breathes effortlessly, and experiences optimal development. Imagine the peace of mind that making informed decisions for your child's well-being brings. This book paints a vivid picture of this better life where the struggles and uncertainties of airway issues are replaced with the joy of watching your child thrive. It enables you to make informed decisions, thus optimizing your child's development and paving the way for a healthier life.

As the author guiding you on this journey, I do not claim authority based on titles or degrees. Instead, my authority comes from the trenches, from battling the same struggles you face today. Although I am not a parent, I was a struggling child and I am a general dentist with a keen interest in orthodontics and a particular focus on treating pediatric patients. My practice embraces the comprehensive dental needs of children, including orthodontic care, to ensure their optimal oral health and development. I understand the challenges, frustrations, and relentless pursuit of answers. Moreover, I understand the lack of accessible information and reluctance of the medical system add complications. This book bridges that gap, consequently providing the missing pieces of the puzzle that can transform your health and your child's airway health. From my experience and research, I have gained quite some information to share.

As you read this book, I want you to feel that it is more than just a guide; it is a companion on your journey. The story within these pages is not just mine; it is a shared narrative of resilience, determination, and the pursuit of a better life for our children. Remember that you are not alone. The struggles, fears, and questions—they are shared by countless parents who have walked this path. Together, let us walk this journey towards a brighter and healthier future.

CHAPTER 1
THE TALE YOUR FACE TELLS

Our early human ancestors actually had dagger-like canines over 4.5 million years ago. This evolutionary change is possibly influenced by female preference for less aggressive partners. Thanks to ancient "dating" preferences, our smiles look a lot friendlier today!

FACES OF THE PAST

The evolution of human facial structure is fascinating. It spans millions of years tracing back to our earliest hominid ancestors. From the primitive features of Australopithecus to the modern characteristics of Homo sapiens, the changes in our facial structure tell a compelling story of adaptation, survival, and evolution.

It all began with Australopithecus who lived around 4 million years ago. These early hominids had protruding jaws, large brow ridges, and a prominent snout-like nose. Their robust facial features were adapted for chewing tough vegetation and foraging in a primarily forested environment—their main source of sustenance.

As time passed and our ancestors transitioned to the Homo genus, their facial structures changed. For example, Homo habilis who dates back around 2.4 million years exhibited a significant reduction in facial prognathism (the protrusion of the lower face). Their faces became flatter and their jaws less robust. This was due to a more varied diet possibly including meat obtained through scavenging.

With the emergence of Homo erectus around 1.8 million years ago, further advancements in facial structure became evident. Their faces were smaller with reduced brow ridges and a more pronounced chin. This change likely reflects advancements in tool use and hunting, as Homo erectus ventured out of Africa and adapted to diverse environments.

The evolution of our own species Homo sapiens marked a significant milestone in facial structure development. Around 300,000 years ago, early Homo sapiens had a high forehead, small brow ridge, and more delicate jaw compared to their predecessors.

As Homo sapiens spread across the globe over the millennia, regional variations in facial structure emerged due to different environmental pressures and genetic adaptations. For instance, populations in colder climates tended to have broader noses to humidify and warm the air, while those in warmer climates often had narrower nasal passages to aid in cooling.

Today, the human face continues to exhibit remarkable diversity. This reflects our rich evolutionary history and the relationship between genetic and environmental factors. Despite these variations, certain fundamental features remain consistent, which emphasizes our shared ancestry as a species.

Effect of Our Lifestyle Changes

The transition from hunter-gatherer to agricultural societies was a significant turning point in human history. It was during this period that our ways of life started changing while simultaneously leaving a lasting imprint on our physical features, particularly our faces. In the days of our hunter-gatherer ancestors, survival depended on skills honed for hunting animals and gathering wild plants. Their faces reflected the demands of this kind of lifestyle with strong jaws and pronounced brow ridges suited for chewing tough foods and withstanding the environment's rigors.

But when agriculture emerged about 10,000 years ago, human societies experienced a significant change. Settlements emerged, and people began cultivating crops and domesticating animals. This altered the way we obtained our food, consequently changing our diet and lifestyle significantly, which in turn influenced the structures of our faces. As agricultural societies developed, reliance on softer, cultivated foods reduced the need for powerful chewing muscles, which led to a decrease in jaw size and a flatter facial profile over generations.

As our ancestors transitioned from the roaming, energetic lifestyle of hunter-gatherers to the more stationary existence of agriculture, their daily physical exertion dramatically decreased. Picture our forebears traversing vast landscapes, relentlessly chasing after fleet-footed prey, and carrying their spoils without any modern conveniences. This intense physical activity not only shaped their bodies but also their facial structures through constant muscular use.

However, with the dawn of agriculture life slowed down. People no longer needed to move as much or as forcefully. This significant drop in physical activity likely influenced changes in facial anatomy, as muscles were not challenged as frequently. Moreover, as farming communities developed, labor became divided with tasks becoming highly specialized. This evolution in societal structure also subtly shifted how people used their facial muscles affecting everything from expressions to social interactions, hence, painted a vivid picture of how our bodies and behaviors adapt to new ways of living.

As these subtle shifts compounded graduall, they resulted in the diverse range of facial features observed in modern human populations.

Impact of Changing Diets on Jaw and Teeth Formation

Throughout human evolution, diets have influenced the anatomy of our jaws and teeth. As our ancestors ate tough and natural foods, their jaw muscles and teeth grew stronger. The act of chewing fibrous and unprocessed food engaged the jaw in a way that stimulated proper development. This explains the nature of the facial features of our ancestors.

With the invention of cooking around 1.9 million years ago—after the discovery of fire—we started eating cooked foods instead of raw food. While this technological advancement made food more digestible, it also changed its texture. Cooked thus softer diets reduced the need for rigorous chewing, which gradually prompted changes in jaw and teeth development. Because the jaws and teeth became less engaged, their size, strength, and robustness reduced.

With more technological advancements in this day and age, we shifted from naturally-cooked to processed foods. This brought about several health issues. The consequences of a shift to softer and processed foods are evident through the increased number of dental health issues. The availability of easily consumable items has contributed to a decline in the natural wear and tear that historical diets once provided. One notable correlation is the rise in dental crowding, as the reduced requirement for aggressive chewing and changed jaw development patterns have been related to misalignments and orthodontic problems in current populations.

In a study by Dr. Weston Price (Price, 1939), poor nutrient absorption interferes with growth and tooth development. He mentioned that the changes in dietary habits are the cause of the emergence of allergies and airway obstruction, which led to mouth-breathing, a shift in tongue posture, and the consequential development of a long and narrow face.

A MAP OF BREATH AND LIFE

The human airway is a complex system comprising various structures that facilitate the passage of air from the external environment to the lungs. The airway is a sophisticated system that consists of the nasal passages, throat (pharynx and larynx), bronchial apparatus (two main bronchi and numerous smaller bronchioles), and lungs. Each of these parts play distinct yet interconnected roles in the process of respiration. From air conditioning and filtration in the nasal passages to gas exchange in the alveoli of the lungs, every component of the airway contributes to maintaining respiratory function and overall health.

Nasal Passages

Your nose is like the air's doorway into your body. This nasal pathway, while simple in structure, is highly sophisticated as it optimizes the air we breathe. Inside the nasal passages, there is a special lining made of mucus and tiny hairs called cilia. The mucus inside the nasal passages moistens the air and warms it up to match our body temperature. This keeps our lungs safe and makes sure they work properly.

The tiny cilia in the nasal passages filter out any dust or dirt particles that try to enter our lungs. They stop these particles from causing any harm and keep our lungs healthy.

There is a wall in the middle of the nasal passages called the nasal septum that splits the space into two parts. This helps the air flow smoothly and does a great job of preparing the air for our lungs. Along the walls, there are three bony shelves called nasal conchae that help with cleaning, moistening, and warming the air we breathe.

These passages are well designed to ensure the air is the right temperature and clean before it reaches our lungs.

Throat

The throat, or pharynx, is a tube at the back of your nose and mouth that helps guide air and food where they need to go in your body. The pharynx is split into three parts: nasopharynx, oropharynx, and laryngopharynx.

First up is the nasopharynx, which connects your nose to your throat and lets air travel smoothly into your respiratory system.

Next, the oropharynx is where your breathing and digestion systems meet and both air and food pass through. It helps air get to your lungs and food go to your stomach when you swallow.

Finally, we have the laryngopharynx. It leads to two important areas: the larynx, which holds your vocal cords for speaking and the esophagus, which carries food to your stomach. The laryngopharynx splits the path for air and food sending air to your larynx for speech and food to your esophagus for digestion.

The larynx, found at the bottom of the pharynx, is like a special box that holds your vocal cords, thus helping you speak. It also has cartilages, like the Adam's apple, that protect your airway. And the epiglottis—a flap of tissue—acts as a gatekeeper during swallowing, hence ensuring food goes down the right way into your stomach and not into your lungs.

Lungs

The lungs help us get the oxygen we need and get rid of carbon dioxide, which is waste. The left and right lung are protected by a special cavity and are split into two and three parts called lobes, respectively, which enables better air movement thus proper breathing.

When we breathe in, air goes through tubes called bronchi and into smaller tubes called bronchioles. These lead to tiny air sacs called alveoli where the magic of breathing happens. In the alveoli, oxygen goes into the blood, and carbon dioxide comes out to be exhaled thus removed.

The alveoli are stretchy, which helps them expand when we breathe in and shrink back when we breathe out. This stretching and shrinking efficiently moves air in and out ensuring proper oxygen supply to and carbon dioxide removal from the body.

Role of the Mouth in Respiratory and Oral Health

The mouth is important in both respiratory and oral health with its various components working together to ensure proper functioning and health. The teeth, tongue, and palate are structures within the oral cavity each contributing significantly to respiratory function, speech articulation, and overall oral health.

Teeth are used in chewing and also in maintaining the integrity of the oral cavity. Properly aligned teeth fit and function in a very specific way, therefore facilitating proper chewing, speech and digestion. This prevents oral health issues like malocclusion (misalignment of the teeth), which affects breathing patterns. Also, teeth provide structural support to the surrounding tissues, including the tongue and palate. This maintains airway patency (the airways ability to remain open) during respiration.

Next, we have the tongue. In addition to its role in taste perception and speech articulation, the tongue is important in maintaining proper oral posture and airway patency. Improper tongue posture such as a low resting position or thrusting against the teeth can lead to malocclusion, obstructive sleep apnea (OSA), and other respiratory issues. But correct tongue posture supports optimal breathing by preventing airway collapse and facilitating nasal breathing, which is essential for proper humidification and filtration of inhaled air.

Then, we have the palate consisting of the hard and soft palate and forming the roof of the mouth. It brings about various benefits related to both respiratory and oral health. The hard palate provides structural support to the upper jaw and teeth, which is important in chewing and speech production. The soft palate is vital for swallowing and preventing food and liquids from entering the nasal cavity, contributes to the modulation of airflow during speech production, and assists in the closure of the nasal passages during swallowing to prevent aspiration.

How Different Components of the Airway Work Together During Breathing

Air's journey begins with the nose and mouth where inhalation starts. These entry points filter, humidify, and warm the incoming air, which protects the delicate respiratory surfaces from potential irritants.

Then, air continues to the throat—a pathway that connects the nasal and oral cavities to the larynx. As air progresses, the larynx—housing the vocal cords—helps regulate airflow and prevents foreign particles from entering the lower respiratory tract. The trachea carries air from the larynx to the bronchi, which ensures a smooth transition.

Branching into bronchi and bronchioles, the air passages further divide and spread throughout the lungs. This branching pattern maximizes the surface area available for gas exchange. The bronchioles lead to the alveoli where oxygen enters the bloodstream and carbon dioxide exits during exhalation.

Surrounding the lungs, the diaphragm and intercostal muscles aid in breathing mechanics (discussed in detail in the next chapter). During inhalation, the diaphragm contracts and moves downward, subsequently expanding the thoracic cavity. Simultaneously, the intercostal muscles between the ribs elevate the rib cage, hence increasing chest volume. This decrease in pressure within the lungs allows air to rush in. Exhalation occurs as the diaphragm and intercostal muscles relax, reducing the thoracic cavity's volume and expelling air as a result.

WHY AIRWAY ANATOMY MATTERS

From the moment of birth to the final exhale, the airway is a lifeline—a complex network of tubes allowing the vital exchange of air. An obstruction in this pathway, whether partial or complete, jeopardizes the flow of life-sustaining air to the lungs—a feeling best avoided. The airway's major role is enabling oxygen utilization in the lungs and nourishing every cell in the body in consequence. A functioning airway ensures cellular growth, cognitive function, and overall bodily movement with breathing being the essence that sustains all bodily systems—from the respiratory and circulatory to the nervous and immune systems.

Breathing is an elemental requirement for life. Unconscious and essential, we take around 500 million breaths in a lifetime, yet seldom contemplate its quality. Emerging scientific evidence emphasizes the impact of airway health on mental and physical well-being, accordingly affecting aspects from sleep to cognitive function.

How Airway Health Affects Sleep Quality

Airway health can determine the quality of your sleep, which influences both the onset and maintenance of a restful night's sleep. Several factors related to airway anatomy and function contribute to sleep quality and disturbances in these areas can lead to the following sleep disorders.

Snoring

Snoring is a prevalent sleep issue that involves soft tissue vibration in the throat caused by airflow obstruction. This obstruction typically occurs as the muscles and tissues relax during sleep causing a narrowing of the air passage. While occasional snoring is normal, persistent and loud snoring can be disruptive not only affecting the snorer but also their bed partner. The constant sound of snoring can lead to fragmented sleep for both individuals resulting in daytime fatigue and a decreased concentration.

Restless Sleep

Restless sleep often stems from airway abnormalities such as nasal congestion or variations in the upper airway structure. Individuals experiencing discomfort due to breathing difficulties may find themselves frequently shifting positions during the night in an attempt to alleviate their discomfort. This constant movement disrupts the continuity of sleep and diminishes its restorative benefits. The restlessness can prevent individuals from entering deeper stages of sleep, therefore impacting overall sleep quality and leaving them feeling fatigued and less rejuvenated upon waking.

Obstructive sleep apnea

OSA is a severe sleep disorder characterized by recurrent episodes of complete or partial airway obstruction during sleep. These episodes lead to momentary pauses in breathing often accompanied by choking or gasping sensations, as the individual's body reacts to the lack of airflow. OSA significantly disrupts the normal architecture of sleep and prevents the affected person from reaching crucial, deeper stages of rest. Consequently, OSA is associated with daytime fatigue, cognitive impairment, and an increased risk of cardiovascular problems.

For example: Emily is a 7-year-old girl who has been struggling with frequent night awakenings. Her parents are concerned about her disrupted sleep patterns and seek medical advice by consulting a pediatrician who specializes in sleep medicine. During the consultation, the pediatrician observes that Emily often breathes loudly and exhibits mouth breathing even during the daytime. The pediatrician suspects that Emily's sleep disturbances may be related to an underlying airway issue. Emily is referred to an orthodontist who specializes in airway-focused treatments. After an examination, the orthodontist diagnoses Emily with a narrow palate and an underdeveloped upper jaw, which can contribute to airway restriction during sleep.

Fatigue

Poor airway health, especially in conditions like OSA, can result in chronic daytime fatigue due to disrupted sleep patterns. The constant interruptions in breathing during sleep prevent individuals from achieving the restorative sleep necessary for optimal functioning. As a result, untreated sleep disorders can lead to daytime drowsiness, poor concentration, and reduced energy, subsequently affecting life quality and productivity.

Insomnia

Airway problems like nasal congestion or breathing difficulties can worsen or cause insomnia. Persistent difficulty falling asleep or staying asleep may arise as individuals struggle to find a comfortable position due to airway-related discomfort. Disruptions in breathing patterns can lead to heightened arousal, thus interrupting the individual's ability to enter sustained periods of restorative sleep. This ongoing sleep disturbance can contribute to chronic insomnia, hence impacting both mental and physical health.

The Link Between Airway Structure and Oral Health

The best and healthiest mode of breathing is through the nose, as it contributes to the proper development of the upper airway and its associated structures. When an obstruction in the upper airway impairs nasal breathing, relying on mouth breathing can lead to several problems associated with airway dysfunction. Mouth breathing is associated with several negative consequences, including the enlargement of tonsils and adenoids. Also, it can contribute to problems such as bruxism (teeth grinding, clenching, or gnashing), teeth fractures, and teeth erosion potentially causing temporomandibular joint disorder (TMD) and myofascial pain.

The habit of mouth breathing may result in malocclusion and impacted teeth disrupting the natural alignment of the jaw, or periodontal disease and an increased risk of dental caries.

QUICK RECAP

- The evolution of facial structure from Australopithecus to Homo sapiens reflects adaptation to changing environments and diets.
- Transition to agricultural societies altered facial features due to changes in diet, lifestyle, and physical activity.
- Dietary shifts throughout human evolution influenced jaw and teeth development leading to dental health issues like dental crowding.
- Airway anatomy impacts oral health with nasal breathing promoting proper development and mouth breathing linked to airway dysfunction and dental problems.
- The human airway consisting of nasal passages, throat, and lungs ensures efficient breathing, conditioning air, and facilitating gas exchange.
- Airway health affects sleep quality with snoring, sleep apnea, and restless sleep being common manifestations of airway dysfunction.

In the next chapter, we will explore the physiological mechanisms behind breathing.

CHAPTER 2
TAKE A DEEP BREATH

On average, infants and toddlers typically breathe 30–60 and 20–30 times per minute, respectively. As people age, this rate generally decreases with older children and adults breathing about 12–20 times per minute at rest. Over the course of a day, this amounts to a staggering 17,000–30,000 breaths. That is a lot of instinctual in-and-outs! This vast amount of breathing occurs seamlessly, which emphasizes the continuous and vital nature of this physiological process at every stage of life.

THE ART AND SCIENCE OF BREATHING

The lower respiratory tract serves as the core of the respiratory system comprising essential components crucial for gas exchange—a vital process that sustains life and maintains cellular function. Key structures within this system include the lungs, trachea, bronchi, and diaphragm. These elements work in concert to facilitate the intricate process of breathing thus ensuring efficient absorption of oxygen and expelling of carbon dioxide with each breath:

- **Lungs:** As the primary organs of the respiratory system, the lungs are responsible for gas exchange. They absorb oxygen from the air we inhale and release carbon dioxide when we exhale. The lungs are spongy, air-filled organs located on each side of the chest.
- **Trachea:** Commonly known as the windpipe, the trachea is a tube that connects the throat to the lungs. It serves as the main airway that allows air to pass in and out of the lungs. The trachea is lined with cilia and mucus to filter out particles and pathogens.
- **Bronchi:** These are the two large tubes that branch off from the trachea into each lung. The bronchi further divide into smaller branches called bronchioles, ultimately leading to the clusters of alveoli. They transport air from the trachea into the lungs.
- **Alveoli:** Tiny air sacs at the end of the bronchial passages, alveoli are where the exchange of oxygen and carbon dioxide actually takes place. Each lung contains millions of alveoli, which are surrounded by networks of capillaries. These structures facilitate the transfer of gases between the lungs and the blood.
- **Diaphragm:** A large, dome-shaped muscle located below the lungs, the diaphragm plays a crucial role in breathing. When it contracts, the diaphragm flattens out, expands the chest cavity, and causes air to flow into the lungs. When it relaxes, the chest cavity

contracts, expelling air from the lungs as a consequence.

The Mechanics of Breathing

The respiratory system is a marvel of biological engineering where various components work in perfect harmony to sustain life through the essential act of breathing. Here is how these parts collaborate to make the magic happen.

Breath Begins

The journey starts with the diaphragm and the chest muscles contracting and pulling downward to create a vacuum that draws air into the body. As you inhale, air travels down the trachea—a sturdy tube reinforced with cartilaginous rings to keep it open as air rushes through.

Branching Out

The trachea splits into two bronchi each directing air into one of the lungs. Inside the lungs, the bronchi branch like the limbs and twigs of a tree into progressively smaller tubes called bronchioles. These pathways ensure air reaches deep into the lungs to every corner and crevice.

The Gas Exchange

Clusters of tiny air sacs called alveoli wait patiently where bronchioles end. Each alveolus is a hub of activity surrounded by a mesh of capillaries so fine and thin that oxygen and carbon dioxide can pass through them. Here in these minute air sacs, the crucial exchange occurs: Oxygen from the air leaps into the bloodstream and carbon dioxide waste jumps out to be exhaled.

The Grand Finale

Once the exchange is complete, the reverse process begins. The diaphragm relaxes springing back to its dome shape, and the chest contracts pushing the spent air back up the bronchial tree, through the trachea, and finally out of the body.

This intricate system is vital not just for breathing but for sustaining every cell in the body. Without this continuous exchange of oxygen and carbon dioxide, cells would not receive the oxygen they need for energy nor could they get rid of carbon dioxide whose accumulation is toxic. The seamless integration of these respiratory parts ensures life continues breath by breath, hence illustrating the beautiful complexity of human biology. Through this delicate balance, we see the interdependent nature of our bodily systems—a reminder of the intricate dance of life happening within us at every moment.

Just as our respiratory structures work together to sustain life, the principles of physics—particularly Boyle's Law—are deeply integrated into the mechanics of how we breathe. This law explains that when we inhale, our diaphragm descends and our ribcage expands, thereby increasing the volume of our chest cavity. This expansion leads to a decrease in pressure within our lungs compared to the external atmosphere, accordingly prompting air to rush in and fill the lungs.

Conversely, exhaling reverses this process: The chest cavity's volume decreases, pressure increases, and air is expelled.

For parents, understanding this interplay between pressure and volume is not just an academic pursuit—it is a critical component of child health care. Recognizing deviations from normal breathing patterns—such as the wheezing in asthma or the labored breathing that may indicate a serious infection—can lead to prompt medical interventions, potentially averting emergencies. Conditions like bronchiolitis, asthma, and pneumonia can impair the lungs' ability to expand and contract, affecting breathing dynamics as a result. Knowledge of these principles helps parents comprehend medical recommendations, including the use of inhalers and other treatments that manage airway pressures.

Moreover, educating children about the science of breathing can cultivate a sense of wonder and curiosity about the human body. Consider the simple joy of blowing bubbles with your child: As the wand dips into the soapy solution and you gently exhale, colorful orbs float into the air. This playful activity is a practical demonstration of Boyle's Law—just as the pressure inside a bubble decreases as it expands, so does the pressure within our lungs when we inhale.

By grasping the physics of breathing, parents not only ensure safer environments but also engage their children in learning experiences that reveal the intricate connections between everyday life and scientific principles. Each time you and your child watch bubbles drift skyward, remember: You are not just creating magical moments, you are exploring the mysteries of the universe one breath at a time.

WHEN FORM MEETS FUNCTION

A healthy and properly structured airway is fundamental to effective breathing. Imagine the airway as the body's grand corridor—essential for the seamless transport of life's breath from the outside world into the inner sanctum of our lungs. This corridor is not just a passive pathway; it is an active, dynamic system lined with vigilant guardians like cilia and mucus that capture and expel invaders such as dust and germs. A well-structured airway ensures that these defenses operate at peak efficiency akin to a well-guarded fortress that keeps the inhabitants safe and healthy.

When this corridor is compromised whether by inflammation, obstruction, or structural anomalies, it is like a bustling market street suddenly clogged with debris. The flow of traffic—air, in this case—slows to a crawl. Each breath becomes a struggle, as if fighting through a crowd on a narrow street while gasping for space. This struggle is not just uncomfortable; it is a direct challenge to the body's ability to perform essential exchanges of oxygen for carbon dioxide, the very transactions that sustain cellular life.

Thus, a healthy and unobstructed airway is not just a convenience; it is critical to the well-being of every organ and cell. It enables the lungs to efficiently convert air into the vital oxygen that fuels every thought, movement, and heartbeat. Keeping this grand corridor clear is not merely about avoiding discomfort; it is about ensuring that life itself can proceed without interruption, hence sustaining every action and dream with each breath we take.

Now, picture your airway as the grand corridor again: Breathing freely should feel like strolling down it—open and unimpeded. However, conditions like asthma can transform this spacious passage into a narrow, constricted tunnel. With asthma, inflammation causes the airways to tighten, much like the walls of a tunnel drawing inwards, turning each breath into a strenuous effort. This leads to symptoms such as wheezing, difficulty breathing, and a feeling of tightness in the chest—clear signs that the once-broad corridor has become a restrictive path.

Adding to this challenge is bronchitis, another affliction that can further complicate the passage through these vital corridors. Like a storm that brings debris and mudslides, bronchitis swells the linings of the airway and fills them with mucus, thus narrowing them even more. This condition not only exacerbates the difficulty of moving air in and out but also triggers a persistent, harsh cough as the body attempts to clear these obstructions.

Allergies too play their role in this complex interplay acting like unexpected gusts of wind that stir up dust and pollen inside this grand corridor. They provoke an overreaction from the body's immune system, which further inflames the airways, creates additional blockages, and intensifies symptoms like sneezing, congestion, and an itchy throat. Together, asthma, bronchitis, and allergies transform this grand corridor into a challenging gauntlet, where each breath becomes a valiant effort to overcome the relentless onslaught of these conditions.

Physical obstructions like tumors act like sudden barriers within this tunnel dramatically narrowing the space and increasing the effort required to push air through. These growths can arise anywhere along the respiratory tract and turn the open passage into a challenging and constricted route. Each breath is now a battle, and the body must work harder for every ounce of air that can leave you gasping and exhausted.

Such obstructions highlight the critical importance of vigilance and proactive health management. Regular check-ups and early detection can be as crucial as maintenance in a tunnel by ensuring it remains clear of flow-disrupting blockages. Just as engineers regularly assess and maintain the integrity of tunnels to prevent collapses and ensure smooth transit, health professionals and individuals must monitor and maintain respiratory health. This approach not only ensures that each breath remains as effortless as possible but also safeguards overall well-being, thus allowing us to navigate the complexities of health with confidence and resilience. Below are several structural differences that can affect breathing.

Deviated Septum

A deviated septum occurs when the nasal septum—the wall between the nostrils—is significantly displaced to one side, subsequently making one nasal passage smaller than the other. This structural irregularity can cause difficulty breathing through the nose, recurrent sinus infections, and nasal congestion. Additionally, a deviated septum can exacerbate snoring and potentially increase the risk of developing OSA.

This condition involves repeated episodes where the airway is partially or completely blocked during sleep leading to disrupted breathing and poor sleep quality. The downstream effect is that it can make you feel fatigued during the day, grumpy, and unable to concentrate. Treatment for a severe deviated septum might involve a surgical procedure known as septoplasty, which straightens the septum to improve airflow and overall nasal function.

Enlarged Adenoids or Tonsils

Adenoids and tonsils are lymphatic tissues located at the back of the throat and nasal cavity, respectively. They play a role in immune function by trapping pathogens entering through the mouth and nose. However, when they become enlarged— possibly due to recurrent infections or genetic predispositions —they can obstruct the airway. This is particularly problematic during sleep as it leads to snoring, sleep apnea, and other breathing disruptions, especially in children. Treatment may involve medication to reduce inflammation or surgery to remove the tissues if they frequently cause breathing or infection problems.

When you or your child face difficulty breathing through the nose, often resulting in frequent mouth breathing, it is crucial to consult with healthcare professionals. This habit can affect more than just breathing; it can also have significant impacts on dental health and facial development. Symptoms like persistent snoring, unusual fatigue during the day, and difficulty breathing could indicate underlying issues, such as enlarged adenoids or tonsils. In these cases, both medical doctors and dental professionals play a vital role. Dentists—skilled in identifying the oral and dental consequences of mouth breathing—can offer essential insights and treatments. Therefore, addressing your concerns with both types of professionals ensures a thorough approach to diagnosing and suggesting ways to help with these health issues.

Tracheal Stenosis

This condition involves the narrowing of the trachea (windpipe) due to inflammation, injury, or a congenital defect. The narrowing can obstruct the airflow, consequently making breathing laborious and noisy. Tracheal stenosis can be life-threatening and may require surgical procedures to widen the trachea and facilitate easier breathing. Doing anything physical makes it worse, as it interferes with catching your breath and doing everyday things.

Cleft Palate or Lip

These are congenital deformities consisting of an opening or split in the upper lip and/or the roof of the mouth that occurs when the facial structures do not fully close during fetal development. Severity ranges from small openings to extensive clefts extending into the nasal cavity. Infants with this condition face challenges—notably breathing difficulties —as the opening may allow air to escape through the nose during feeding, speaking, or breathing and possibly lead to significant problems with feeding, speaking, and breathing. Additionally, individuals with cleft palate or lip are at higher risk of ear infections due to structural abnormalities affecting

Eustachian tube function—the opening that connects the middle ear with the nasopharynx—potentially impacting hearing. Speech development is hindered by structural variations that affect sound formation, articulation, and language development. Speech therapy and surgery are often recommended to address these challenges and improve functionality.

Nasal Polyps

These are soft, painless, noncancerous growths on the lining of the nasal passages or sinuses. They result from chronic inflammation and can be associated with asthma, recurrent infections, allergies, or certain immune disorders. Nasal polyps cause long-term congestion that hinder breathing through the nose and cause constant stuffiness. They disrupt airflow and scent detection therefore making breathing uncomfortable during activity or exercise and reducing the ability to enjoy smells, respectively. Large polyps can obstruct the nasal passages and lead to breathing difficulties, a reduced sense of smell, and frequent infections.

BREATHING TROUBLE: SIGNS TO WATCH IN CHILDREN

Sometimes, you may see children who seem to have a hard time breathing when they are playing sports, enjoying outdoor activities, or even just relaxing. About 4.2 million children globally suffer from asthma and other respiratory conditions and face challenges that range from mild discomfort to severe, life-threatening difficulties.

It is not uncommon to hear about children who need hospital care because they cannot stop coughing, or to know someone who misses school for extended periods due to breathing issues. Breathing difficulties can be painful and sometimes disrupt taking a deep breath. As a result, they might find it tough to participate in favorite activities like sports or spending time with friends, which is truly disheartening. Witnessing a child struggle for breath can be distressing for everyone around.

At the core of these issues are various pediatric respiratory disorders—from the wheezing of asthma to allergy-induced sneezes and coughs that often signal infections. Let us discuss the spectrum of these conditions to understand their nuances and impacts on our young ones.

Asthma

Imagine a world where every breath is a struggle, where simple pleasures like running in a park could suddenly turn into a daunting battle for air. Asthma—marked by a reversible airway inflammation and tightening of its surrounding muscles—transforms this grim scenario into daily reality for many children and makes each breath a laborious task. This condition does not discriminate against triggers—smoke, pollen, or even a faint whiff of perfume can set off a cascade of symptoms including wheezing, coughing, and an oppressive chest tightness. If not well-managed, asthma can escalate to severe complications; statistics show that about one in 20 asthmatic children are hospitalized each year. However, with diligent care, proper medication, and strategy, these young warriors can manage their asthma effectively and enjoy lively, active days just like their peers but always with a watchful eye.

Allergies

Picture a battlefield where everyday elements become foes. For children with severe allergies, everyday substances like pollen, pet dander, or a simple dusty shelf trigger defensive reactions from their immune systems, subsequently causing a barrage of uncomfortable symptoms: relentless sneezing, itchy, watering eyes, and a runny or congested nose that seems endless. Nearly one in five children deal with these challenges, and for many these allergic reactions are compounded by asthma making every breath a struggle. About 19% of children suffer from allergies, and there is a notable overlap with asthma—eight out of 10 children with asthma also battle allergies exacerbating their respiratory symptoms. Allergy management not only involves antihistamines and avoiding known allergens but also includes educating peers and teachers about potential triggers and responses. This network not only helps mitigate the immediate allergic reactions but also fosters a broader understanding of how deeply these conditions can affect a child's life—from school attendance to social interactions and emotional well-being.

Infections

When typical cold symptoms escalate into severe health threats, children's smaller airways become dangerous battlegrounds. Illnesses like croup and respiratory syncytial virus (RSV) transform ordinary coughs and fevers into severe medical ordeals accompanied by the distinctive, harsh sounds of a barking cough or alarming wheezes. These infections target the very young particularly hard, as the small size and anatomical proximity of their airways to their Eustachian tubes predispose them not only to more severe breathing difficulties but also to painful ear infections. The onset of cooler months heightens these risks, as infections become more rampant and the air itself can aggravate their tender airways. Proactive and preventative health measures, thorough hygiene practices, and timely medical intervention are crucial to shield these vulnerable young bodies from the potentially devastating impacts of these infections.

Congenital or Structural Problems

From their very first breath, some children are confronted with extraordinary challenges. Conditions such as cystic fibrosis create a relentless reality where thick, sticky mucus clogs their lungs, thus severely hindering their ability to breathe and progressively impairing lung function.

According to the Cystic Fibrosis Foundation, about 40,000 children are battling this condition as their pulmonary strength slowly erodes over time. Other young individuals may struggle with chronic lung conditions characterized by lesions, scarring, or swelling—each breath a labor, each day a testament to their vulnerability. Yet, there is hope in the form of meticulously crafted care plans, which include cutting-edge medications, specialized breathing therapies, and sometimes innovative surgical solutions. Each condition demands a specialized approach from a team of healthcare professionals —from pediatricians to pulmonologists and surgeons—all dedicated to help enable these children to embrace each day with renewed strength and hope.

Symptoms and Signs Indicating Potential Breathing Issues in Children

Children who struggle with breathing might show signs that they are not getting enough oxygen, a condition that can escalate into respiratory distress. Recognizing these signs early is crucial in managing potential health risks effectively.

If your child is breathing faster than usual or if you notice a bluish tint around their mouth, lips, or fingernails, it might indicate that their body is craving more oxygen. Pale or grayish skin is another warning sign that should not be ignored. Listen for any grunting noises as your child breathes out—this could mean their body is working overtime to keep their airways open and prevent their lungs from collapsing.

Observe your child's breathing closely. Do their nostrils flare when they inhale? Does their chest seem to retract around the neck, breastbone, or ribs? These are signs that they are struggling to pull in enough air. A sweaty head and cool, clammy skin might also indicate that their breathing rate has increased.

In situations where oxygen is lacking, you might see your child's neck muscles straining or their head bobbing with each breath signaling a serious effort to breathe. Loud, harsh sounds when inhaling could point to an obstruction in the upper airway while a tight, whistling, or musical sound during breathing suggests narrowed air passages—common in conditions like asthma or bronchitis.

Early detection and treatment of respiratory issues are paramount. Catching these signs promptly allows for swift medical intervention, which can prevent the condition from worsening. Timely medical care not only aids in symptom management but also helps ensure that your child's lungs continue to function optimally.

Effective treatment is key in managing respiratory problems. Early diagnosis enables you to choose the most appropriate interventions whether that involves medication, lifestyle adjustments, or specialized support programs designed to improve lung health. Initiating treatment early greatly enhances its effectiveness.

Prompt attention to respiratory concerns is vital to prevent severe complications. Ignoring these signs can lead to dire consequences, such as severe breathing difficulties or even cardiac issues. Early intervention not only minimizes the risk of serious complications but also improves your child's overall health and quality of life, hence allowing them to enjoy more vibrant and joyful days despite their respiratory challenges.

QUICK RECAP

- Breathing rates vary across ages reflecting age-dependent respiratory patterns: infants breathe at 30-60 breaths/minute, toddlers at 20-30 breaths/minute, and adults at 12-20 breaths/minute.
- Critical respiratory components include the lungs, trachea, bronchi, alveoli, and diaphragm, which enable efficient gas exchange necessary for sustaining life.
- Breathing mechanics follow Boyle's Law, governing air pressure changes during inhalation and exhalation. Inhalation involves diaphragm contraction and rib elevation, while exhalation is driven by muscle relaxation i.e., passive.
- Airway structure and function are maintained by nasal passages, pharynx, larynx, trachea, bronchi, and bronchioles ensuring efficient airflow. Structural variations like asthma, tumors, or infections can obstruct airflow leading to breathing difficulties.
- Structural issues such as deviated septum, enlarged adenoids, tracheal stenosis, cleft palate, or nasal polyps can impede breathing, accordingly underscoring the importance of early detection and intervention for improved outcomes and quality of life.

The next chapter will focus on the role of early childhood development in shaping facial structure and airway health.

CHAPTER 3
GROWING UP WITH A HEALTHY SMILE

Babies often start sucking their thumb in the womb as a natural reflex and a way to self-soothe. It is one of the first coordinated actions a baby can do that demonstrates an innate ability to seek comfort and manage stress from the earliest stages of life. In rare cases, the habit of thumb sucking can persist into adulthood often as a hidden behavior used for stress relief. This seemingly innocuous action is more than just a cute milestone; it is actually an important sign of how natural instincts and physical growth are connected. While it is normal for babies to suck their thumbs, doing it persistently can lead to unexpected problems with a child's facial development, dental alignment, and airway health. So, paying attention to this habit helps us understand what babies need emotionally and highlights how early habits can significantly impact their health as they grow.

FOUNDATIONS OF A HEALTHY FACE

The human face is truly remarkable, as it is composed of more than 40 muscles that work together harmoniously. These muscles offer a wide range of functions: from simple tasks like breathing to more complex actions like expressing emotions. They enable us to convey feelings through facial expressions like smiling, frowning, and countless others. In early childhood, the bones of the face and jaw grow rapidly thus setting the foundation for adult facial structure. Humans have different types of tissues in the body each with specific characteristics and functions. Hard tissues provide structural rigidity and support, while soft tissues play roles in support, movement, and various physiological functions.

Hard Tissue Profile Changes

Skull

When babies are born, their skulls are soft and flexible. The skull is made up of many bones that are separated by soft spots called fontanelles. These fontanelles act like little hinges that allow the skull to flex slightly during birth, which makes it easier for the baby to exit the birth canal. They also give room for the baby's brain to grow quickly in the early stages.

As the baby grows, its skull bones start to harden and come together—a process called cranial ossification. It begins at the fontanelles and then to the rest of the bones, making the skull stronger as a result. The skull is mostly fused together by the age of two, although some parts might take longer to fully connect.

Having a properly developing skull during infancy is important because it ensures there is enough space inside the head for essential structures such as the brain and airways. The size and shape of the skull affect the size of the airway, how the mouth grows, the alignment of the teeth and the development of the jaws. Importantly, improper development of the skull leads to airway issues. For example, craniosynostosis—premature fusion of the skull bones —can result in restricted skull growth leading to craniofacial abnormalities and airway obstruction.

During infancy, skull development is influenced by the baby's positioning and movement. Activities such as tummy time, crawling, and reaching encourage the natural growth and shaping of the skull because they promote muscle strength and coordination. You should also ensure proper positioning of the baby to prevent conditions like positional plagiocephaly —a flattening of one side of the skull that can occur when infants spend excessive time in a single position, such as lying on their backs.

Jaw Development

Babies' skulls continue developing from infancy to childhood, especially in the area of the face. This development includes changes in the bones of the upper (maxilla) and lower (mandible) jaw. These changes create space inside the mouth for teeth and ensure they line up properly. When the child has a well-developed jaw, they are more likely to have enough room for correct positioning of all teeth.

During this stage, their jaws go through a lot of changes, especially when their baby teeth fall out and are replaced by permanent ones. This change influences oral health and the functionality of their airway. The timing and order of the new teeth's appearance can impact how the jaws grow and the teeth line up. If a child loses its baby teeth too early because of issues like cavities or accidents, it can lead to crowded teeth and malocclusion due to loss of space for permanent teeth when this happens. The child who develops properly aligned teeth is more likely to have an open airway and optimal oral health.

Proper jaw growth in children is influenced more by their environment than by genetics, so even if you and your partner have certain jaw shapes, it does not guarantee your child will inherit them. The upper jaw undergoes significant growth by the age of nine or 10, while the lower jaw continues to develop into the teenage years dependent on the surrounding muscles and tissues. Proper alignment of these parts is crucial as it impacts breathing, facial appearance, jaw joint health, and how the teeth fit together. By actively guiding the growth of the upper jaw and addressing any muscular issues, you can enhance your child's overall health. This proactive approach can lead to a broad, happy smile with straight teeth, potentially reducing the need for braces in the future.

Nasal Cavity Development

A significant feature of the face is the nose, which is primarily made up of soft tissue. Typically, an infant's nose is short and round with a button-like appearance. Initially, a baby's nose is quite small, but it grows larger as it ages to allow more air intake. It is positioned relatively low on the face with an inward-curving bridge and nostrils that are visible from the front. The infant's nose does not protrude much and is not very long vertically.

As the children grow up, their nasal cavities go through a series of changes that affect how they breathe. Their nose keeps growing and changing along with the rest of their face. What is actually fascinating is that our noses continue to grow in our late teens or early twenties even after we have stopped growing in height. While other parts of our body reach their full size at the end of adolescence, the nose keeps growing steadily at a rate of about 1–1.3 mm per year until we reach adulthood.

As the face develops, the palate changes shape to fit with the rest of the face. Certain habits, such as prolonged thumb sucking, may cause some children to develop a high-arched or narrow palate further constricting the airway.

This narrowing can complicate breathing, particularly during sleep, similar to the issues that arise when the skull, jaws, and nasal cavity do not grow properly. These irregularities can lead to crowded teeth, malocclusions, and significant breathing difficulties. In cases where the upper or lower jaw is underdeveloped, the airway may become restricted and increase the risk of sleep apnea. Moreover, misaligned teeth or an inadequately developed palate can disrupt the normal airflow through the nose, subsequently exacerbating these respiratory challenges.

Soft Tissue

Oral Cavity

Key components in the development of soft tissues include the tongue, tonsils, and lips. First, let us talk about the tongue, which is made up of a few different muscles. Your tongue might seem small, but it is actually pretty strong and it pushes on the roof of the mouth with every swallow. Correct swallowing involves the tongue applying approximately 500 g of weight to the roof of the mouth and stimulating nerves and blood vessels that trigger the pituitary gland to release pleasure-inducing hormones. Inadequate swallowing techniques can hinder the natural production of these hormones, potentially resulting in the development of behaviors like thumb sucking or the reliance on pacifiers to cope.

It is a really busy muscular organ too, as it assists in swallowing about 1,200–2,000 times each day. Your tongue's position in your mouth matters a lot. When you are not eating or talking, it should naturally rest on the roof of your mouth. If it does not, it can push against your teeth and change how they grow resulting in crowded or flared out teeth.

Having your tongue in the right spot helps your upper jaw grow nicely and enhances your facial appearance. But sometimes, breathing through your mouth, keeping it open, or having a tongue tie can change how your tongue sits inside the mouth. An open mouth pulls the tongue backward, potentially blocking the air passage and disrupting jaw development. This can lead to crowded teeth and a less defined facial structure due to inadequate pressure from the tongue on the jaw. So, make sure your tongue rests in the right place.

However, sometimes people develop a habit called tongue thrusting where the tongue pushes against the teeth or sticks out between them when swallowing. This habit can cause problems like misaligned teeth and difficulties with speech.

Now, what are tonsils? Tonsils, often overlooked but crucial to our health, are clusters of tissue located at the back of the throat. They act as the body's first line of defense against harmful pathogens by trapping bacteria and viruses. Additionally, tonsils play a vital role in the immune system, producing antibodies that help ward off future infections. However, when tonsils become enlarged, they can pose a serious risk to breathing. Large tonsils can obstruct the airway leading to breathing difficulties, particularly during sleep. If a child exhibits symptoms such as loud snoring, pauses in breathing during sleep, or difficulty swallowing, it is imperative to seek the expertise of an ENT doctor for assessment. Timely intervention and management of enlarged tonsils are essential to ensure unimpeded breathing and overall well-being.

As a parent, ensuring the proper development of your child's face and jaw from a young age is paramount. One common habit that can adversely affect this development is thumb-sucking, which we need to address carefully.

CURBING DETRIMENTAL HABITS EARLY

Whether they realize it or not, many babies are fascinated with sucking their thumbs from the moment they first learn about their fingers and toes. Perhaps you even brought home a blurry picture of your unborn child contentedly self-soothing from an ultrasound scan when you were pregnant.

Getting your child to stop sucking their thumb seems as easy as persuading them that the blue cup is equally as excellent as the red one. They are only three or four years old; it is not going to be that easy.

Besides thumb-sucking, there is pacifier use and bottle feeding. The impact of thumb sucking, pacifier usage, and bottle feeding on facial development holds considerable importance, especially during the critical phases of development in infancy and early childhood.

The American Academy of Pediatrics has some rules about using pacifiers. They say it is satisfactory for babies to use pacifiers when they sleep to help prevent sudden infant death syndrome (SIDS) but only after the baby has gotten used to breastfeeding, which is usually when they are about 3–4 weeks old. Also, premature use of pacifiers is discouraged because it could make breastfeeding difficult. It is important to use a clean pacifier that is all one piece and not attach anything like ribbons or strings because it becomes a choking hazard. You should also check the pacifier often for any damage and replace it if needed for safety. While pacifiers can help comfort babies, it is important to use them the right way by following these guidelines.

Bottle feeding, especially when continued for an extended period, can also impact facial development. The sucking motion required during bottle feeding can affect the muscles involved in jaw movement. Improper bottle-feeding techniques or reliance on bottles for an extended duration may contribute to malocclusions, as well as impact the overall muscular balance in the face.

As a parent, you should intervene early when you notice that your child does them by using the following strategies.

Thumb-Sucking

Encouraging your child to break the thumb-sucking habit is ultimately their decision, but as a parent you can adopt various strategies to support them in this process. Positive reinforcement, praise, and rewards have proven to be effective tools for some parents.

If your child is ready to kick the habit, here is a step-by-step guide on weaning toddlers or preschoolers. Begin by preparing your child, introducing the concept, and discussing the reasons behind the decision with them.

Taking a gradual approach is crucial. Designate a specific location, such as their bed where thumb-sucking is allowed, while discouraging the behavior in other parts of the house. Weaning the child slowly is best at bedtime by allowing thumb-sucking only then.

Positive reinforcement can greatly motivate your child. Rather than continuously pointing out the undesired behavior, focus on praising them when they refrain from thumb-sucking. Implementing a reward system, such as stickers or extra bedtime stories, and tracking progress on a calendar can reinforce their success.

Providing alternatives is another strategy. When you observe thumb-sucking, offer activities that keep their hands occupied like a fidget toy or a stress ball. Try to find alternative ways of comfort, such as using a stuffed animal or other objects.

Teaching new coping skills is essential, as children may suck their thumbs to cope with emotions like fear or anxiety. Identifying triggers and helping them practice mindfulness, breathing exercises, listening to music, or engaging in kid-friendly yoga can replace thumb-sucking as a coping mechanism.

Recognize when professional help is needed. Extreme measures like applying bitter substances on the thumb may upset children, and it is important not to eliminate their coping strategy prematurely. Consult your child's healthcare provider or dentist if you have concerns about their thumb-sucking habit, as early identification can be crucial for resolution. In some cases, a dentist may recommend a dental appliance or a thumb guard to discourage thumb sucking by making it less satisfying or comfortable.

Pacifier

Below are some alternative strategies for helping your toddler give up their pacifier:

1. Reduce pacifier use by clearly defining when it is appropriate, such as only during sleep or when feeling stressed.
2. Practice patience-building exercises and deep breathing with your child daily to help them learn self-calming techniques without relying on the pacifier.
3. Set designated "pacifier-free" periods during the day to gradually reduce dependence. Start with short intervals and use a timer to enforce the rule gently.
4. Boost your toddler's confidence by whispering praises to their stuffed animals about their pacifier-free achievements.
5. Gradually wean them off by trimming the pacifier's nipple over time until it is a small nub, then present it to your child by gently explaining that it is broken and cannot be used anymore.
6. Incorporate stories into your routine about characters who successfully part ways with their pacifiers while emphasizing the positive feelings associated with letting go.
7. Avoid telling your toddler that the pacifier will be given to another baby, as it might create jealousy. Instead, consider imaginative explanations such as sending it to a magical place.

8. Involve your child in choosing a special day to bid farewell to the pacifier by marking it on a calendar with stickers and counting down together.
9. Offer an exchange where your toddler receives a new toy or reward in return for giving up the pacifier, thus making the transition more enticing.

Keep a cheerful attitude throughout the process and avoid placing pressure on your child. Every child develops at their own pace, so be patient and helpful even when setbacks arise.

Bottle Feeding

Before transitioning your child from bottles to cups, it is important for them to learn how to drink from a cup. Pediatricians recommend introducing sippy cups to children between 6–9 months of age, which aligns with the period when babies may begin to explore water and other beverages beyond breast milk or formula. This transition coincides with the World Health Organization's (WHO) guidance that all infants be exclusively breastfed for the first six months to gain essential nutrients and antibodies necessary for optimal growth. As babies approach this age, they can also start to try complementary foods that introduce them to a variety of textures and tastes, hence fostering healthy eating habits and aiding in the development of oral motor skills. Parents should watch for signs of readiness for these new experiences around the 6-month mark and consult their pediatrician to ensure the introduction of appropriate foods and drinking methods.

Starting early with offering milk in cups rather than solely relying on bottles can make the eventual transition smooth. Straw sipping can be offered at the same time, but not pushed if the baby does not catch on to it.

When you are ready to stop using bottles altogether, there are two main approaches: going cold turkey or gradually weaning off. Both methods have their challenges with cold turkey being the quickest but potentially the toughest emotionally for parents.

Whether you choose to go cold turkey or wean slowly, expect some resistance from your child. Resistance is normal and should be anticipated regardless of the approach you take.

With the cold turkey method, you remove all bottles abruptly. Involving your child in the process by explaining the transition to them can help ease the change.

Weaning involves gradually replacing bottles with cups starting with one feeding per day and gradually increasing. You can begin with mid-day bottles first, followed by the morning one, and finally tackle the nighttime bottle.

Removing the nighttime bottle tends to be the most challenging step, as it can disrupt bedtime routines and make it harder for both parents and babies to sleep. Establishing a consistent bedtime ritual, such as a warm bath, reading a story, and cuddling with a comfort item, can help soothe your child without relying on the bottle.

Baby-Led Weaning

A method of introducing solids by focusing on infant self-feeding and serving the family's table foods is called baby-led weaning (BLW). It may begin around six months, when the baby shows signs of readiness such as sitting up independently, loss of tongue thrust reflex, mouthing toys, and showing interest in table foods. There are many sample food charts available online to try that offer guidance and inspiration for parents embarking on the journey of baby-led weaning.

Self-feeding is a key component of BLW and provides babies with many opportunities to develop and practice both gross and fine motor skills. Exploring and picking up foods on their own increases the number of opportunities babies have to practice strength-building movements, therefore fostering the development of essential motor skills.

Introducing babies to different textures and tastes involves both a sensory and chewing component, and there is a critical window of time for this exploration. Without exposure to varied textures and tastes, children may develop aversions and become selective eaters. Transitioning from purees to solid foods can be challenging with concerns about choking often at the forefront of parents' minds. However, gagging during this transition could be indicative of underlying issues such as myofunctional disorders or a tongue tie which causes difficulty manipulating food in the mouth. Additionally, the adenoids or tonsils could be obstructing the airway. In such cases, seeking assessment from healthcare professionals including doctors, dentists, ENT specialists, speech language pathologists (SLPs), or myofunctional therapists is essential for proper diagnosis and intervention. By addressing these concerns early on, parents can ensure their child's healthy development and enjoyment of diverse foods.

THE BRAIN-BITE CONNECTION

Oral Motor Disorder

An oral-motor disorder means there are problems with the muscles in the mouth and throat that can make eating, talking, and swallowing difficult. These problems come in three main types. Oral or verbal apraxia is when someone cannot move their mouth the way they want to usually because their brain has trouble planning the movements. A second oral disorder is dysarthria, which happens when it is hard to eat safely or talk clearly often because of mouth and throat muscle weakness. If the muscles needed for eating do not develop correctly, it can cause trouble with chewing, swallowing, and handling food properly. These issues need careful checking by a doctor and specific treatments to help improve these functions and overall oral health.

Additionally, low muscle tone in the lips, tongue, or jaw can contribute to oral-motor disorders manifesting as difficulties with specific mouth movements. These challenges may become apparent during meal times such as struggles with manipulating food, using a straw, or excessive drooling, which are indicative of potential lip or tongue weaknesses.

Recognizing these signs early is crucial and consultation with a pediatrician should be the initial step.

Speech Language Pathology

A referral to a SLP may follow for a specialized evaluation since they are experts in diagnosing and treating these disorders. When checking for oral-motor disorders, the SLP will talk to you about what you have noticed at home and will also check your child in different ways. They will look for any weakness or poor muscle control in your child's lips, jaw, and tongue; watch how your child copies movements that are not related to talking; see how well their muscles work together when they try to speak; test how your child does in normal and pretend activities. This detailed check-up helps the SLP understand your child's needs better, subsequently allowing them to develop a special plan that includes various therapeutic techniques and exercises aimed at improving muscle strength, coordination, and control in the mouth and throat. This plan is tailored to help your child use their mouth muscles more effectively.

Working on certain speaking and eating activities during therapy can help a child get better at these skills over time. Progress in developing these skills can vary greatly; it may be gradual and influenced by the nature of the challenge, child's engagement, and frequency of practice within the family setting; conversely, it can be remarkably swift. With hard work and support from both the therapist and the family, kids with oral motor problems can really get better at eating, talking, and communicating. Regular check-ups with the speech therapist will help keep track of the child's progress and make changes to the therapy plan if needed to maintain improvement.

Myofunctional Therapy

Myofunctional issues in children can lead to various physical and social challenges. These issues may manifest in different ways indicating the potential need for myofunctional therapy.

Difficulties with food and eating such as sensitivity to textures, picky eating, or gagging can indicate swallowing challenges, particularly during the transition to solid foods. Speech development may also be affected evidenced by delayed speech or articulation issues, potentially indicating tongue positioning problems or tongue-tie that may require a frenectomy.

Certain habits like prolonged pacifier use or thumb-sucking may exacerbate myofunctional issues leading to improper tongue posture and swallowing patterns, ultimately impacting facial growth. Myofunctional issues can disrupt sleep by causing sleep apnea, snoring, or bedwetting, which may result in behavioral problems resembling attention deficit disorder/attention deficit hyperactivity disorder (ADD/ADHD) due to poor sleep quality.

Moreover, incorrect jaw positioning such as overbite or underbite may signal underlying myofunctional issues affecting facial and dental development. Children with myofunctional issues may experience frequent ear infections and enlarged tonsils or adenoids due to mouth breathing, hence emphasizing the importance of addressing swallowing problems to mitigate associated health concerns.

Initiating myofunctional therapy early can help correct problems before they become more severe and may reduce the need for surgeries, such as tonsillectomy or adenoidectomy. This therapy includes a series of exercises designed to strengthen the facial, oral, and tongue muscles, consequently targeting issues that affect speaking, eating, and breathing. By tackling these foundational problems, myofunctional therapy promotes a child's growth, development, and especially elimination of the need for habits like thumb sucking or pacifier use.

Children as young as 4 or 5 can begin myofunctional therapy, but the starting age may differ based on the child's needs. Consulting a qualified therapist is crucial to assess your child's situation and determine the ideal time to begin therapy.

In myofunctional therapy, the goal is to promote and sustain correct oral habits, such as

- encouraging nasal breathing
- ensuring the lips come together naturally when not in use
- promoting an upward resting position of the tongue against the palate
- enhancing awareness of proper chewing and swallowing patterns

IT IS TIME FOR FACIAL FITNESS!

When aiming to support your child's facial development, SLPs and myofunctional therapists will engage them in practical exercises. These exercises not only aid in enhancing facial appearance but also contribute to the improvement of their oral motor skills. Here is why engaging in facial exercises is important:

- **Improves muscle tone:** These exercises strengthen facial muscles crucial for eating, speaking, and facial expressions.
- **Enhances articulation skills:** Strengthening the muscles of the lips and tongue is crucial for speech, as it leads to improved mouth movement, clearer pronunciation, and better understanding.
- **Helps in clear speech production:** Targeted exercises, especially for the lips and tongue, aid in controlling airflow during speech and promoting clearer expression.
- **Oral motor skills development:** Strengthening and coordinating cheek muscles support various oral activities beyond speech, therefore enhancing overall oral health and function.

By doing these exercises with your child, you are not only helping them look and feel better but you are also setting them up for success in their communication skills. These exercises include:

- **Blowing bubbles**: This is for lip and cheek weakness but it is fun, and kids will play with bubbles without even knowing it is therapy.
- **Using straws to drink:** Drinking from straws strengthens a child's lip and cheek muscles, thus aiding in tongue positioning and creating a mature swallowing pattern. It is advisable to introduce straw cups by the age of one to encourage these developments.
- **Making funny faces:** Imitating funny faces—depending on your child's weakness—alongside chewing exercises for toddlers will both entertain and help.
- **Lollipops:** Yes, they can be used in therapy. Your therapist will have your child lick the lollipop or different candies using its tongue in different positions so that the tongue gains strength. Doing tongue exercises for speech therapy is very important.

QUICK RECAP

- Thumb sucking often starts in infancy and can persist into adulthood as a stress reliever.
- Early childhood is critical for facial and jaw bone growth, as it shapes adult facial structure.
- Notable changes include forehead size reduction, nasal bone evolution, and mandible growth.
- Soft tissue profile changes, such as nose and lip growth, influence facial aesthetics.

- Parents play a vital role in fostering healthy oral habits and facial development.
- Facial fitness exercises improve oral motor skills and speech clarity.
- Myofunctional therapy addresses physical and social issues in children starting from age 4 or 5.

In the next chapter, various breathing exercises will be discussed.

CHAPTER 4
BREATHING RIGHT

In children under eight years old, the prevalence of mouth breathing is about the same as nose breathing. After they turn eight, however, approximately 35% of children without allergies or obvious nasal obstructions continue to breathe primarily through their mouths.

THE POWER OF PROPER BREATHING

The power of proper breathing cannot be overstated when it comes to your overall health. It is not just about inhaling and exhaling; it is about doing it correctly and intentionally to reap the maximum benefits for your body and mind.

First and foremost, proper breathing techniques are vital for enhancing oxygenation in your body. Deep and full breaths allow more oxygen into your bloodstream, hence fueling every cell, tissue, and organ. This body fuel energizes you, improves stamina, and boosts vitality. It is like giving your body a refreshing boost of vitality with each breath.

Moreover, proper breathing is intimately linked with improved concentration. When you are stressed or anxious, your breathing tends to become shallow and irregular, which can hinder your ability to focus. However, by practicing deep, diaphragmatic breathing, you activate your parasympathetic nervous system, subsequently promoting relaxation and mental clarity. This allows you to concentrate better on tasks at hand whether it is studying for an exam, tackling a work project, or simply being present in the moment.

Further, proper breathing techniques are a powerful tool for managing stress. Stress is an inevitable part of life, but how you respond to it can make all the difference in your well-being. Deep breathing induces the body's relaxation response, countering stress hormones such as cortisol and adrenaline as a result. It slows down your heart rate, lowers your blood pressure, and induces a sense of calmness and tranquility. When you add deep breathing exercises into your daily routine, you can develop resilience to stress and maintain a greater sense of equilibrium amidst life's challenges.

In addition, proper breathing improves sleep quality by calming the mind and nervous system. Relaxation techniques such as deep breathing before bedtime signal your body to unwind and promote peaceful sleep. This helps reduce insomnia and restless sleep, which are often caused by stress or racing thoughts. Thus, deep breathing leads to feeling refreshed in the morning and prepares you for the day ahead.

So, how does effective breathing impact physical and mental health? When you breathe effectively, you provide your body with the oxygen it needs to function optimally. This benefits your physical health by ensuring that your organs and muscles receive enough oxygen to operate efficiently. It also significantly improves your mental well-being. Deep and steady breathing can help calm your mind, reduce stress levels, and promote relaxation.

Casual and Mindful Breathing

There are two main ways one can breathe: casually and mindfully. Casual breathing is automatic—performed without conscious thought—and simply sustains life by delivering oxygen to the body with minimal effort. It continues regardless of whether you are busy, resting, or stressed as your body manages this vital function on its own. When you breathe casually, you do not pay much attention to the process; it is primarily about survival.

Mindful breathing, on the other hand, involves a deliberate focus on each breath. Rather than breathing absentmindedly, you concentrate on the sensations of inhaling and exhaling. This practice helps you stay present, hence shedding distractions and easing worries. You may observe the movement of your belly or chest, or the air flowing through your nostrils. Mindful breathing is not only about relaxation but also serves as an effective tool for managing stress and anxiety. It allows you to detach from negative thoughts and emotions, thereby fostering greater balance in your life. With regular practice, mindful breathing becomes a natural self-care habit.

While casual breathing is essential for basic survival, mindful breathing enhances your awareness and peace of mind. It taps into a hidden well of calm and energy that can enrich your daily life.

NASAL MATTERS

Nasal and mouth breathing are two primary methods by which humans intake air. The key difference lies in the pathways through which air enters the respiratory system.

When you breathe through your nose, the air passes through small passages before reaching your lungs. Inside your nose, tiny hairs and moist membranes clean, warm, and moisten the air. This process filters out dust and other particles to ensure that the air is safe for your lungs. Additionally, your nose adjusts the air's temperature to match your body's, which is particularly beneficial in cold or dry environments.

On the other hand, when you breathe through your mouth, the air travels directly in and out without passing through the nose. People often breathe through their mouths when their noses are blocked or when they consciously choose to do so. Unlike nose breathing, mouth breathing does not clean or warm the air, which means it can be colder and drier by the time it reaches your lungs. This can increase your likelihood of getting sick or experiencing irritation in your throat or lungs. Sometimes, mouth breathing occurs due to factors like allergies or nasal obstructions that make it difficult to breathe through the nose.

Besides the physical sensation of the air, the way you breathe also influences your stress and relaxation levels. Breathing through your nose can help you relax because it activates the parasympathetic nervous system, which is responsible for the body's "rest and digest" response. On the other hand, breathing through your mouth might make you feel more stressed and anxious, as it is associated with faster, shallower breaths that stimulate the sympathetic nervous system known for triggering the "fight or flight" response.

Breathing through your nose enhances health in several key ways beyond the basic functions of air filtration and moisturizing. It increases the production of nitric oxide, which not only improves blood flow but also bolsters the immune system and keeps the heart functioning efficiently. Additionally, it promotes deeper, more relaxing breaths contrasting with the stress-inducing and less oxygen-efficient mouth breathing. Furthermore, nasal breathing helps prevent dry mouth and bad breath by maintaining moisture in the oral cavity.

Habitual Mouth Breathing

This refers to consistently breathing through the mouth instead of the nose, which poses significant health risks. It causes dryness in the mouth and throat, which can be uncomfortable and may lead to irritation, as the warming and moisturizing roles of the nose are not utilized.

Moreover, such breathing habits adversely affect oral health. Prolonged mouth breathing can lead to dental issues such as cavities, gum disease, and misaligned teeth, which may require orthodontic treatment. A drier mouth means less saliva to protect your teeth, allowing more harmful bacteria to grow thereafter.

So, why is saliva a superhero for your mouth? It plays a crucial role by neutralizing acids, enhancing tooth remineralization, and protecting against infections—all essential for maintaining oral health. It contains a variety of substances that contribute to these functions. A key component includes bicarbonate, which acts as a natural neutralizer to balance acid levels.

Additionally, saliva contains calcium and phosphate crucial for strengthening tooth enamel and lysozyme—an enzyme that attacks harmful bacteria. It helps control the microbial population in your mouth by inhibiting bacterial growth and protecting against oral infections. Also, an antibody called immunoglobulin A (IgA) is present, which aids in immune defense. Proteins in saliva, including mucins and histatins, play multifunctional roles. Mucins help clear bacteria and viruses from the mouth and lubricate oral tissues hence alleviate chewing and swallowing food. Histatins provide antimicrobial properties and aid in wound healing. Together, these substances work to protect teeth and gums, prevent decay, and ensure a healthy oral environment.

Maintaining both the quality and quantity of saliva are essential for maintaining oral health; insufficient saliva production or altered saliva composition can increase the risk of cavities. Additionally, a reduction in saliva—often due to mouth breathing—can lead to enamel erosion, thus increasing tooth decay and sensitivity. This issue of reduced saliva flow is particularly concerning at night, as it may exacerbate or be indicative of conditions like sleep apnea that causes disrupted breathing during sleep and can further impair saliva production and overall oral health.

Breathing through your mouth while sleeping can lead to issues such as snoring and sleep apnea. These disturbances not only disrupt sleep but also contribute to health problems like cardiovascular issues and daytime fatigue. Additionally, mouth breathing can exacerbate oral health problems such as bruxism (teeth grinding) and influence facial aesthetics in children, potentially resulting in a longer facial structure and a less defined jawline.

Maintaining a proper lip seal where the lips comfortably rest together without strain promotes healthier nasal breathing and is superior to mouth breathing, as it filters and warms the air, improves oxygen exchange, and maintains moisture levels. This is crucial for preventing dry mouth, which can lead to dental decay and gum disease. A consistent lip seal also supports optimal facial development and proper teeth alignment, eventually enhancing both aesthetic appearance and speech clarity through improved articulation and sound production.

WHY THE LONG FACE?

Long face syndrome—a high-arched palate, narrow upper jaw (maxilla), underbite (retrognathia), and an elongated lower facial section—predominantly affects children who prefer mouth breathing over nasal. This habitual mouth breathing alters the harmonious development of facial bones and muscles leading to aesthetic and functional changes.

The syndrome's onset is often linked to a mix of environmental and genetic factors, including chronic nasal congestion, allergic reactions, and structural irregularities within the nasal passages. These factors disrupt the natural downward and forward growth of the jaw, accordingly steering facial development toward a more vertical orientation. The term "long face syndrome" encapsulates these changes by highlighting the significant impact of breathing habits on facial structure from an early age.

Connection Between Breathing Patterns and Long Face Syndrome

The link between how we breathe and the shape of our faces is key to understanding long face syndrome. Normally, nasal breathing helps shape the face evenly and ensures that the jaws and facial muscles develop correctly. But when someone breathes through their mouth instead, it can lead to a stretched-out look in the face—a sign of long face syndrome. Mouth breathing can change the way the tongue rests, which then affects the way the upper jaw grows. Things like constant allergies or large tonsils can impede nasal breathing, which can cause more frequent mouth breathing and negatively impact how their face grows.

The Health Implications of Long Face Syndrome

The ramifications of long face syndrome extend far beyond cosmetic concerns deeply influencing overall health and well-being. Dental issues are prevalent with misaligned teeth and jaws complicating basic functions like chewing, speaking, and increasing susceptibility to oral health problems. The altered facial structure can lead to narrowed airways and escalate the risk of sleep apnea—a condition linked to serious health issues like hypertension, heart disease, and cognitive impairments.

The psychological impact of the syndrome cannot be overlooked, as the visible changes in appearance may lead to a diminished self-image and quality of life. Addressing these complex challenges requires a multidisciplinary treatment approach including orthodontic care, surgical interventions, and targeted therapies to correct breathing patterns aiming to restore both function and confidence.

BREATHEEASY 360 METHOD

Understanding the effects of poor breathing habits like those seen in long face syndrome underscores the importance of adopting correct breathing techniques early in life. Transitioning from these issues, the BreatheEasy 360 Method presents a comprehensive solution that not only counteracts poor habits but enhances overall health through its holistic approach to breathing.

The BreatheEasy 360 Method is a deep breathing technique that optimally uses the diaphragm and other respiratory muscles to foster full-body health. This method, named for its ability to expand the ribs and torso in a complete circle (360°), ensures that breathing is not limited to the front body —like the chest or abdomen—but includes the side ribs and back as well. This comprehensive expansion aids in more than just respiration; it also influences posture and internal organ function.

Although it might seem complex, 360 breathing is actually a return to the natural breathing patterns we have as infants that are lost as we age due to stress, prolonged sitting, and inactivity. By relearning to breathe deeply, not only can we alleviate physical tension and pain in areas like the neck and shoulders but we can also activate the diaphragm more effectively. This activation is crucial, as it enhances the function of core and pelvic floor muscles—areas often weakened by modern lifestyles.

The process of 360 breathing can be broken down into three distinct phases for clarity and ease of practice:

1. **Diaphragmatic breathing:** Your diaphragm contracts and moves downward expanding the abdomen and pelvic floor.
2. **Rib cage expansion:** Your rib cage expands laterally and posteriorly allowing your lungs to fill more completely with air.
3. **Back body expansion:** This phase involves the expansion of the back of the torso, which not only relaxes tight back muscles but also supports spinal alignment and core muscle strength.

Implementing the 360 breathing method brings numerous benefits that extend across various aspects of health and well-being. Regularly practicing this technique enhances the respiratory system by strengthening the breathing muscles and increasing lung capacity, which ensures a more efficient oxygen intake and overall vitality. This method is especially beneficial for stress management; by promoting deep and rhythmic breathing, it activates the parasympathetic nervous system i.e., reduces stress and induces relaxation. This relaxation is crucial for achieving restorative sleep, thereby improving sleep quality and contributing to overall mental health.

For children, the developmental advantages are particularly significant. Proper breathing techniques are essential for normal facial and dental development by helping prevent issues related to improper jaw alignment and growth, such as those seen in long face syndrome. Additionally, enhanced breathing mechanics improve respiratory efficiency by enabling airway clearance and lung protection, especially in environments laden with pollution or allergens.

BREATHING EXERCISES FOR THE LITTLE ONES

Teaching breathing exercises to toddlers brings substantial benefits to both their emotional and physical growth. These techniques help toddlers manage their emotions by providing them a way to calm themselves during moments of distress or excitement, which is crucial as they face more complex social situations. Enhanced focus and concentration are additional benefits—essential as they begin structured educational activities like preschool. On the physical side, these exercises improve oxygen exchange, boost energy levels, and strengthen the immune system—key for young children building their defenses against illness. They also promote better sleep by helping toddlers relax before bedtime and ensuring they get the necessary rest for healthy development. Moreover, incorporating fun activities like bubble blowing or feather floating not only engages toddlers but also aids in developing fine motor skills and body awareness, therefore establishing early habits for a lifetime of good health and emotional balance.

Bubble Blowing or Straw Blowing

Blowing through a straw or blowing bubbles is a fun and effective way for children to strengthen their breathing muscles and improve breath control. Show them how to inhale deeply through their nose, and then exhale slowly through the straw or bubble wand while focusing on prolonging their exhalation. Engage them in playful activities like blowing cotton balls across a table or creating bubbles, which makes learning enjoyable.

Feather Floating

Feather floating is a playful and effective exercise for teaching toddlers control over their exhalation. Provide your toddler with a light feather or a piece of fabric and have them try to keep it in the air by blowing air slowly and steadily. This activity not only keeps them engaged through the gentle floating of the feather but also helps them learn to regulate their breath's strength and speed.

Balloon Breath

Balloon breath is an engaging and simple exercise designed to help children learn the fundamentals of deep breathing in a fun and relatable way. To begin, have your child sit comfortably with a straight back. Instruct them to inhale deeply through their nose while imagining they are filling up a balloon inside their belly. Encourage them to hold their breath for a short moment to maximize the feeling of fullness. Then, they should slowly exhale through their nose while visualizing the balloon deflating. This visual aid helps children grasp the concept of controlled breathing. Repeat this process for a few minutes, as you remind your child to maintain slow and deep breaths.

Flower and Candle Game

This is a simple and engaging way to teach toddlers breath control. Begin by providing a visual aid, such as a pretend flower or a real one with an appealing scent. Encourage your child to inhale deeply through their nose and imagine the process of smelling the flower. Then, guide them to exhale slowly through their mouth as if they are gently blowing out a candle. This playful approach not only makes the learning process enjoyable but also effectively helps them understand how to modulate their breathing.

BREATHWORK FOR SCHOOL-AGE KIDS AND TEENS

For older school-age children and teens, integrating breathing exercises into daily routines can have profound effects on their well-being and academic performance. These exercises are particularly beneficial in reducing mouth breathing, which often leads to dental issues and poor sleep quality. By training the body to inhale through the nose, these practices not only filter and humidify the air but also utilize the nasal passages' natural defenses against pathogens. Regularly performing these techniques during calm periods, such as in the morning or before bedtime, helps manage stress and anxiety while improving concentration and mental focus. Continuous practice will improve respiratory efficiency and help maintain proper dental and facial structure by supporting natural growth patterns encouraged by nasal breathing.

As students navigate the complexities of school life and social interactions, breathing exercises serve as powerful tools for stress management and emotional regulation. They help older kids and adolescents stay calm and composed during tests, presentations, and other high-pressure situations. Physically, deep breathing increases oxygen flow to the brain, thereby enhancing concentration and mental clarity. Moreover, it promotes relaxation, reduces symptoms of anxiety and depression, and improves sleep patterns—game-changers during the stressful teenage years. To maintain these benefits, it is crucial for teens to make these exercises a consistent part of their lifestyle and consider engaging in activities like yoga, which further emphasize breath control. Educators and parents can support these efforts by participating themselves, demonstrating the exercises' benefits, and encouraging a routine practice.

Diaphragmatic Breathing

This is deep and slow breathing using the diaphragm. Start by finding a comfortable position either lying flat with a pillow under your knees or sitting upright in a chair with your knees bent. Place one hand on your upper chest and the other just below your rib cage on your belly. Inhale slowly through your nose making sure your stomach expands against your lower hand, while the hand on your chest should remain relatively still. Hold the breath for a brief moment, about 2–3 seconds, and then exhale slowly through pursed lips while tightening your abdominal muscles to aid the exhalation. Ensure the hand on your stomach moves inward as you exhale. Repeat this process for several minutes, as you concentrate on the movement of your abdomen. Regular practice of this breathing technique, ideally for 5–10 minutes at least once or twice daily, can significantly improve your respiratory efficiency and aid in stress management.

4-7-8 breathing

The 4-7-8 breathing technique, developed by Dr. Andrew Weil, is a simple yet powerful exercise designed to promote relaxation and stress relief. Initially, it is best to perform this technique while seated with a straight back, but you can also practice it lying down as comfort increases. Place the tip of your tongue just behind your front teeth and against the roof of your mouth. Begin by exhaling completely with a "whoosh" sound to empty the lungs. Then, inhale quietly through your nose for a count of four. Hold your breath for seven counts, thereby allowing the oxygen to absorb into your bloodstream. Finally, exhale completely with a "whoosh" sound for eight counts. This pattern helps regulate the nervous system, therefore reducing anxiety and improving sleep.

Square Breathing

The "square breathing" technique, or "box breathing," is a practical and effective method for focusing your thoughts and alleviating stress, particularly after challenging situations. To practice this technique, you will need a piece of paper and drawing tools, or you can simply visualize a square with your eyes closed. Begin at the bottom left corner of the square by inhaling deeply as you draw the line upward to the top left corner. Hold your breath as you continue drawing the line across to the top right corner. Then, slowly exhale as you move the pen down to the bottom right corner. Finish by holding your breath once more as you draw the line back to the starting point at the bottom left corner. This rhythmic pattern of breathing and drawing helps stabilize emotions and syncs movement with breath, therefore enhancing your ability to calm both mind and body effectively.

Bhramari Pranayama (Bee Breathing)

Bhramari Pranayama, also known as the bee breathing technique, is a calming yoga practice that involves humming during exhalation to produce a soothing sound similar to that of a buzzing bee. This exercise is renowned for its ability to relieve stress, reduce anxiety, and calm the mind. A quiet place to sit comfortably in with your eyes closed is of utmost importance. Then, taking a deep breath in through your nose would be your second step. As you exhale, gently close your ears with your thumbs, and place your index fingers on your forehead and your remaining fingers over your eyes. Then, make a loud humming or "hmmm" sound from your throat while feeling the vibration throughout your head. This vibration helps to soothe the nervous system and promote relaxation. Repeat this process for several breaths, ideally 5–10 times, to maximize its calming effects. Regular practice of Bhramari Pranayama can improve concentration, alleviate migraines, and enhance overall mental wellness, accordingly making it a valuable addition to any daily meditation or yoga routine.

Alternate Nostril Breathing

Alternate nostril breathing, also known as Nadi Shodhana, is a calming and balancing pranayama technique. To practice this method, position your right hand by bending the pointer and middle fingers into your palm and leaving the thumb, ring finger, and pinky extended. Start by finding a comfortable seated position and close your eyes or softly gaze downward. Take a moment to inhale and exhale deeply to prepare. Begin the breathing cycle by using your thumb to close off your right nostril, and inhale slowly through the left nostril. After inhaling, use your ring finger to close the left nostril, then release the right nostril and exhale smoothly. Continue by inhaling through the right nostril, then close it with your thumb, and exhale through the left nostril to complete one full cycle. This practice is especially beneficial before stressful activities or as part of a regular meditation practice.

QUICK RECAP

- Proper breathing is essential for overall health.
- Deep and intentional breathing enhances oxygenation throughout the body.
- Proper breathing aids in improving concentration and mental clarity.
- Deep breathing techniques are effective for managing stress and promoting relaxation.
- Proper breathing promotes better sleep quality and aids in stress management.
- Nasal breathing is superior to mouth breathing for overall respiratory health.
- Breathing through your mouth can cause dental issues and trouble sleeping.
- Long face syndrome can result from habitual mouth breathing and has significant health implications.
- Breathing exercises tailored to different age groups can help improve breathing habits and reduce stress.

In the next chapter, we will discuss the influence of lifestyle factors on airway health, and you will understand how everyday habits impact breathing and learn strategies to improve respiratory health through lifestyle changes.

MAKE A DIFFERENCE WITH YOUR REVIEW
UNLOCK THE POWER OF GENEROSITY

Money can't buy happiness, but giving it away can.

FREDDIE MERCURY

People who give without expecting anything in return live longer, happier lives and often find more success. So if there's a chance we can help each other during our time together, I'm all in.

To make that happen, I have a question for you...

Would you help someone you've never met, even if you never got credit for it?

Who is this person, you ask? They are like you. Or, at least, like you used to be. They want to make a difference, need help, and aren't sure where to start.

Our mission is to make improved airway development accessible to everyone. Everything I do stems from that mission. And the only way for me to accomplish that mission is by reaching...well...everyone.

This is where you come in. Most people do, in fact, judge a book by its cover (and its reviews). So here's my ask on behalf of a struggling parent or healthcare professional you've never met:

Please help that parent or healthcare professional by leaving this book a review.

Your gift costs no money and takes less than 60 seconds to make real, but it can change a fellow parent's or healthcare professional's life forever. Your review could help…

...one more small business provide for its community.
...one more entrepreneur support their family.
...one more employee find meaningful work.
...one more client transform their life.
...one more dream come true.

To get that 'feel good' feeling and help this person for real, all you have to do is...and it takes less than 60 seconds...

leave a review.

Scan the QR code below:

If you feel good about helping a parent or healthcare professional, you are my kind of person. Welcome to the club. You're one of us.

I'm that much more excited to help you achieve optimal airway health easier than you can possibly imagine. You'll love the strategies I'm about to share in the coming chapters.

Thank you from the bottom of my heart. Now, back to our regularly scheduled programming.

- Dr. Markus Wilson

PS - Fun fact: If you provide something of value to another person, it makes you more valuable to them. If you'd like goodwill straight from another parent or healthcare professional - and you believe this book will help them - send this book their way.

CHAPTER 5
LIFESTYLE CHOICES THAT COUNT

Many of us have attempted to improve our posture by pulling our shoulders back and down, but did you know this common quick fix might be doing more harm than good? This approach can destabilize your shoulder joints and strain your neck. Because it is an unnatural and tiring position to maintain, it often leads us right back to slouching. So, what is a better way to enhance our posture without these drawbacks?

POSTURE AND BREATHING

Good posture, characterized by a straight back and open chest, enhances breathing by allowing full and effective lung expansion and diaphragm function. This optimal alignment aids in deep, efficient breathing. On the other hand, poor posture such as slouching or hunching compresses the chest and impedes the diaphragm's movement resulting in shallow breaths and reduced oxygen intake. Continuous poor breathing habits can lead to fatigue, decreased lung capacity, and other respiratory problems.

Effects of Slouched Position

To avoid any negative effects, it is crucial to be conscious of maintaining proper posture throughout the day. This practice ensures that your breathing is not compromised, thereby supporting better lung function and reducing the risk of respiratory issues. Regularly adjusting your position and incorporating stretches or exercises that strengthen back and shoulder muscles can help sustain good posture and enhance your overall well-being.

An example is how our digital habits are reshaping our physical health like the increasing prevalence of "tech neck," a modern epidemic of poor posture driven by our growing reliance on smartphones and computers. This condition develops when frequent downward glances at screens lead to structural issues in the back and neck as well as respiratory difficulties. In this strained posture, neck and shoulder muscles must work overtime to support the head, consequently becoming tight and sore while the back muscles weaken from their efforts to maintain an upright position. This not only restricts deep breathing but also heightens feelings of fatigue and anxiety, hence highlighting the profound impact of our digital lifestyles on our physical well-being.

What Are the Consequences of Shallow Breathing?

Shallow breathing, marked by quick, superficial breaths, exacerbates health issues significantly. When your breaths are shallow, your body fails to receive adequate oxygen leading to feelings of fatigue, dizziness, and mental fog. This inefficient breathing pattern triggers a stress response causing your heart rate to spike and muscle tension to increase, especially around the neck and shoulders. Over time, this can lead to weakened muscles, diminished lung function, and elevated stress and anxiety levels.

In stark contrast, deep abdominal breathing sends a powerful calming signal throughout the body, fostering relaxation and reducing stress as a result. Deep breathing-promoting techniques like mindfulness not only bolster physical health but also enhance mental well-being By mastering and incorporating deep breathing practices, you can effectively counteract the negative consequences of poor posture and shallow breathing, ultimately enriching your quality of life.

STAND TALL

Ensuring your child maintains proper posture while sitting is crucial for their overall body health and strength. When seated, encourage them to sit up straight, push their shoulders back, and place their bottom deep in the chair to maintain the spine's natural curve. This posture not only distributes their weight evenly—reducing strain on any single part of the body and preventing back pain—but also promotes better breathing and concentration.

Does good posture really matter at their age? Why do they need good posture?

Did you know that maintaining good posture can increase lung capacity by up to 30%? Proper alignment promotes efficient breathing by allowing the chest to expand fully, which optimizes lung function and enhances oxygen intake. This improvement in respiratory efficiency boosts overall health, mood, and energy levels making daily activities and learning both more enjoyable and productive. To encourage children to maintain good posture, consider incorporating fun and engaging methods such as posture checks or a reward-based scoring system especially at meal times.

Furthermore, good posture is essential for avoiding common discomforts like back pain and headaches. It minimizes strain on muscles and joints, thereby enhancing overall comfort. Additionally, maintaining proper posture improves visual motor skills, which are crucial for precise tasks like writing neatly and performing well in sports. In physical activities, correct posture enhances balance, agility, and power while also reducing the risk of injuries. It also promotes better spatial awareness and coordination leading to increased self-confidence and more positive social interactions.

How to Improve Your Child's Posture

When you incorporate these tips into your child's daily routine, you can help improve their posture and set them up for a lifetime of good spinal health.

- **Be the example**: Demonstrate good posture by maintaining an upright stance with shoulders back and head high. Children naturally mimic their parents, so your consistent example is a powerful, silent lesson in the importance of good posture.
- **Encourage barefoot walking**: Walking barefoot engages and strengthens the muscles in the feet, ankles, and legs. This not only supports the arches but also improves overall body alignment and balance, thus teaching your child to adjust their posture naturally.
- **Ensure aligned furniture**: Provide ergonomically designed furniture that supports good posture. Chairs should offer adequate back support and desks should be at a height that allows your child to keep their spine neutral while seated. This setup helps in developing and maintaining correct posture habits during study and work.
- **Choose the right backpack**: Opt for a backpack that fits well and evenly distributes weight across the shoulders. A backpack with padded straps and multiple compartments can minimize the load on any single point of your child's back, therefore aiding in correct posture and preventing any potential discomfort.
- **Teach proper eating habits**: Encourage your child to sit up straight while eating, which involves bringing the food to their mouth rather than bending forward. This not only aids digestion but also helps in maintaining a healthy posture by reducing strain on the neck and spine.

- **Take frequent breaks**: Regular breaks from sitting or screen time are crucial. Encourage your child to get up and stretch at least every hour. This breaks the monotony of prolonged sitting and promotes better posture, circulation, and muscle flexibility—essential for overall spinal health.
- **Incorporate movement**: Promote an active lifestyle with activities like sports, yoga, or dancing. Regular movement helps build core strength and flexibility—essential for supporting a healthy spine and joints. Active habits also help mitigate the negative effects of excessive sitting and lead to better posture as your child grows.

By implementing these strategies and providing ongoing encouragement and positive reinforcement, you can help your child develop and maintain good posture for a healthier future.

GET MOVING

Physical activity plays a crucial role in enhancing respiratory health notably by strengthening the muscles involved in breathing i.e., the diaphragm and intercostal muscles. Engaging in activities that increase heart rate—running, swimming, or playing sports—not only strengthens these muscles but also improves lung capacity. This allows for deeper, more efficient breaths and enhances the ability of the lungs to expand and contract. Interestingly, the diaphragm—the primary breathing muscle—can become significantly stronger through aerobic exercises, thus promoting better oxygen intake.

Moreover, exercise boosts cardiovascular health, which in turn increases the blood flow to the lungs. This enhanced circulation helps the body utilize oxygen more effectively, energize muscles, and improve overall endurance. Activities that involve consistent deep breathing, such as jogging or brisk walking, are especially beneficial as they train the lungs to handle larger volumes of air i.e., increase respiratory efficiency.

Adding to the variety of ways to boost respiratory health, high-altitude training offers a unique method for enhancing lung function. When athletes train at high altitudes, they do so in environments with lower oxygen levels. This challenging setting compels the body to adapt by increasing red blood cell production and improving oxygen utilization efficiency. Such adaptations can significantly boost endurance and respiratory capacity even when the athlete returns to sea level, hence showcasing the body's remarkable ability to adjust and optimize lung function under varied conditions.

Certain exercises, like yoga or targeted breathing drills, specifically focus on lung flexibility and capacity. These activities help maintain the elasticity of the lungs, thereby ensuring optimal functioning through prevention of respiratory ailments and ensuring the longevity of lung health. Regular physical activity is also instrumental in managing and alleviating symptoms of respiratory conditions such as asthma or chronic obstructive pulmonary disease (COPD). By fortifying the respiratory system and improving cardiovascular function, exercise can reduce symptoms like shortness of breath and wheezing, which makes it a vital component of respiratory health management.

Integrating regular exercise into daily routines is essential for both preventing and managing respiratory issues. Encouraging your child to engage in simple, regular exercises such as cycling, jumping rope, or even playful running games can be a fun and effective way to help them develop strong respiratory and cardiovascular systems.

The Rocker

Begin by sitting on the floor with your knees bent and feet flat. Grasp your shins with your hands and lean back slightly until you are balancing on your sit bones. Carefully lift your feet off the ground aiming to bring your shins parallel to the floor. Balance in this position by actively engaging your core muscles to stabilize your body. Hold this pose for a few seconds to challenge your balance and strengthen your abdominal muscles. Gently lower your feet back to the floor to return to the starting position. Repeat this movement for several repetitions while focusing on maintaining smooth, controlled movements throughout the exercise. This pose is excellent for enhancing core strength and improving balance.

Wall Angel

Begin by standing with your back flat against a wall and feet set hip-width apart. Make sure your lower and upper back and head are pressed firmly against the wall. Extend your arms out to shoulder height and bend your elbows at 90° angles keeping your palms facing forward. Gradually slide your arms upward along the wall reaching as high as possible without allowing your back to arch or your arms to come off the wall. Then, carefully slide your arms back down to the starting position. Repeat this movement for several repetitions. This exercise is excellent for improving posture and strengthening the shoulder muscles while ensuring the spine remains aligned.

Butterfly Wings

Begin by sitting on the floor with the soles of your feet pressed together and your knees bent outward to each side. Grasp your ankles with your hands to stabilize your posture. Ensure your spine is straight as you sit up tall, then gently use your elbows to press your knees toward the floor, thus enhancing the stretch in your inner thighs and lower back. Hold this position for a few seconds to deepen the stretch, then release gently. Repeat the stretch several times while focusing on maintaining a tall, straight posture and moving smoothly to maximize the benefits to your hips and back. This exercise is great for improving flexibility and reducing tension in the lower body.

Tight Rope

Start by standing tall with your feet together and extending your arms to the sides to help maintain balance. Visualize yourself walking on a tightrope. Begin walking forward with slow, deliberate steps while focusing on maintaining a straight line. Keep your gaze fixed on a point directly in front of you to aid in balance. As you walk, engage your core and concentrate on keeping your posture upright. After taking several steps forward, carefully turn around and walk back to your starting point. This exercise helps improve balance, coordination, and core strength making it ideal for enhancing body awareness and stability.

Tilting Star

Start by standing with your feet hip-width apart. Extend your arms overhead with your palms facing each other. Then, lean to one side as you stretch the arm on that side over your head while bending your torso toward the opposite side. Keep your feet firmly planted and your core engaged to help maintain balance. Hold the stretch for a few seconds while feeling the elongation along your side. Return to the upright starting position, then repeat the stretch on the other side. Continue alternating sides for several repetitions. This stretch is excellent for enhancing side body flexibility and improving overall balance.

Downward-Facing Dog Yoga Pose

Start by positioning yourself on your hands and knees with hands and knees set shoulder- and hip-width apart, respectively. Push firmly through your palms and gradually lift your hips up toward the ceiling while extending your arms and legs as you go. Aim to keep your back straight and your heels pushing down towards the floor, although it is okay if they do not fully touch. Hold this pose for a few deep breaths while concentrating on lengthening your spine and distributing your weight evenly through your palms. After holding, gently return to the starting position. This pose helps stretch and strengthen various parts of the body while calming the mind.

Animal Walks

Start by selecting a specific animal movement such as bear crawls, crab walks, or frog hops. Position yourself on all fours for bear crawls or on your hands and feet with your stomach facing up for crab walks. For frog hops, start in a crouched position. Mimic the chosen animal's movement pattern as you traverse across the floor, simultaneously ensuring your back remains straight and your core engaged to maintain proper posture. Experiment with various speeds and styles to target different muscle groups and add a playful yet challenging element to your workout that enhances muscular strength, flexibility, and coordination.

Superman

To execute the Superman exercise, begin by lying flat on your stomach with your arms extended in front of you and your legs straight behind. Engage your back muscles to simultaneously lift your arms, chest, and legs off the floor. Ensure your gaze is directed downwards to keep your neck in a neutral position. Hold this elevated position for a few seconds to maximize engagement in your lower back and glutes. Then, carefully lower yourself back to the starting position. Repeat the movement several times while focusing on smooth, controlled motions and maintaining form to strengthen the back and improve posture.

Bridges

Start by lying on your back with your knees bent and your feet flat on the floor, positioned hip-width apart. Pressing firmly into your heels, lift your hips upward until your shoulders, hips, and knees form a straight line. As you raise your hips, engage your glutes and tighten your abdominal muscles to support your lower back. Hold this position for a moment before gently lowering your hips back down to the floor. Repeat this movement several times, focusing on maintaining form and steady breathing throughout the exercise. This pose is excellent for strengthening the core, glutes, and lower back.

These exercises engage various muscle groups, enhance posture, and boost overall strength and flexibility in children. Encourage your children to include these exercises in a fun and healthy routine. For older kids and teens, exercises such as side plank, high plank, chest opener, standing cat-cow, forward fold, and child's pose are also beneficial. Chapter 8 will provide detailed explanations of each exercise through exploring their benefits and proper techniques. Incorporating these exercises into a teenager's routine can improve flexibility, strengthen muscles, and promote better posture during critical growth periods.

QUICK RECAP

- Good posture enhances lung capacity and breathing mechanics by facilitating efficient diaphragmatic movement and proper spine alignment.
- Slouching impedes diaphragmatic function and contributes to shallow breathing, while tech neck exacerbates breathing difficulties and musculoskeletal issues.
- Shallow breathing reduces oxygen intake leading to fatigue and stress while also causing muscle tension and impaired respiratory function.
- Good posture reduces strain on muscles and joints, improves visual motor skills, and enhances sports outcomes.
- Be a posture role model, encourage barefoot walking and aligned furniture, incorporate movement to strengthen respiratory muscles, and promote better posture through various exercises.

In the next chapter, you will learn the link between nutrition, oral and airway health, and the dietary guidelines that support oral health and improve breathing.

CHAPTER 6
CHEW ON THIS

Lily, an 8-year-old patient, sits nervously in the dentist's chair, her small frame barely filling the space. Despite her parents' diligent efforts with regular brushing, Lily's weak enamel and multiple cavities puzzled me. As I examined Lily's teeth, I gently asked about her eating habits. Lily's parents shared their concern, revealing Lily's penchant for sugary snacks and drinks, especially her favorite candy, gummy bears, and soda. My heart sank as I realized the impact of Lily's diet on her dental health. This pivotal moment vividly illustrated the critical importance of nutrition in maintaining oral health. Lily's story is the gateway to a broader discussion within the chapter exploring the critical link between nutrition, oral health, and airway health.

YOU ARE WHAT YOU EAT

Nutrition plays a crucial role in maintaining oral and airway health by providing the essential nutrients needed for the development and upkeep of the mouth and airways. A balanced diet rich in various foods supplies essential vitamins, minerals, proteins, and nutrients necessary for optimal health. For oral health, this diet is integral to the well-being of teeth, gums, and the structural integrity of the mouth and airways.

Key nutrients such as calcium and phosphorus—found in dairy products, leafy greens, nuts, and seeds—are essential for building strong teeth and bones. Vitamin D enhances calcium absorption—crucial for forming tooth enamel and preventing decay. Additionally, vitamin C—abundant in fruits and vegetables like oranges, strawberries, and bell peppers—supports gum health by aiding collagen production, which keeps gums resilient and less susceptible to disease.

Nutrition also influences the facial structure, particularly the development of the jaw and airways, ensuring clear airways and optimal breathing. Proteins from meat, fish, eggs, and beans are vital for the growth and repair of facial muscles and bones, therefore supporting proper jaw alignment and airway function.

Moreover, a balanced diet prevents oral health issues by limiting intake of harmful sugars and acids found in candies and sodas. These substances foster bacterial growth leading to plaque, decay, and enamel erosion, which can result in tooth pain and decay. By prioritizing a balanced diet, you can safeguard your oral and airway health, thereby ensuring a stronger, healthier mouth and clearer breathing pathways.

Role of Nutrition in Shaping Our Facial Structure

Our dietary choices—significantly different from the diets of our ancestors—play a critical role in the development of our palates. Modern diets, often rich in refined and processed foods, do not provide the necessary stimulation for proper growth. This can lead to dental and respiratory issues over time. Historically, diets that required extensive chewing helped develop stronger jaw muscles and more robust palates.

Incorporating raw fruits and vegetables into your diet is crucial for proper palate development. These foods demand more chewing, which in turn stimulates jaw muscle activity and encourages full development. Additionally, including calcium-rich foods like almonds, kale, and salmon enhances bone health, which is essential for the development of the palate and teeth.

Dietary fats, along with fat-soluble vitamins such as A, D, E, and K2 are vital for holistic growth and bone formation. Vitamin A—crucial for bone health and immune function—is abundant in carrots, sweet potatoes, and spinach. Vitamin D— important for calcium absorption and bone growth—can be sourced from fatty fish like salmon, fortified dairy, and sunlight exposure. Almonds and sunflower seeds are excellent sources of vitamin E, which supports skin health and immune function. Vitamin K2, found in fermented foods like natto, certain cheeses, as well as in egg yolks is essential for bone metabolism and cardiovascular health. These nutrients together play a comprehensive role in ensuring a well-developed palate and overall health.

The Consequences of Poor Nutrition on Dental Health and Facial Development

Imagine a child's plate filled with typical favorites like pizza and fries. This seemingly innocent meal could be subtly influencing their future respiratory health. Research suggests that the Western diet—rich in processed foods and saturated fats—may double the risk of developing asthma by age four. This striking statistic highlights how crucial early dietary choices are, potentially setting the stage for a lifetime of wheezes and sneezes.

Now, think about a child's penchant for sweets. Each sugary treat is not just a delight to their taste buds but also a feast for harmful bacteria in their mouth. These bacteria thrive on sugar, produce acids that erode teeth, and lead to cavities that can compromise a child's beautiful smile. But there is more to strong, healthy teeth than avoiding sweets and just brushing. Nutrients like calcium and vitamin D found abundantly in leafy greens and dairy are essential. They do not just strengthen bones; they fortify teeth, thus protecting them from becoming as fragile as old chalk.

By turning our kitchens into battlegrounds for good health and equipping our children with nutrient-rich foods, we are not just filling bellies; we are launching a lifetime of good health and beautiful smiles. Encouraging a diet rich in essential nutrients and limiting processed and sugary foods can dramatically influence their overall health. This is not just about avoiding illness; it is about promoting vitality and well-being that can last a lifetime.

How Nutritional Deficiencies Can Impact Facial Symmetry

Nutritional deficiencies can disrupt how evenly balanced the features on each side of a person's face are leading to facial asymmetry. When someone does not get enough essential nutrients, one side of their face can look slightly different from the other. For example, one eye might be a bit higher or larger or one side of the mouth might be wider. These differences are usually small and not very noticeable.

Fluctuating asymmetry describes these small differences between the left and right sides of the face, which result from random developmental mistakes. This means the person's appearance slightly strays from their ideal genetic blueprint. Unlike changes caused by genetics or environment, these subtle variations simply show that no two sides of any face are perfectly identical.

What are the causes of poor facial symmetry? Three major factors play pivotal roles: nutrient deficiencies, improper breathing, and bad posture.

Imagine the face as a canvas where nutrients paint the broad strokes of symmetry. When essential elements like vitamins, minerals, and proteins are scarce, the painting becomes unbalanced. Lack of calcium and vitamin D, for instance, is like missing strokes on this canvas leading to uneven bone growth and resulting in a face where one side may not quite match the other—perhaps one cheekbone stands out more or the jawline slants subtly.

Improper breathing, especially mouth breathing, also significantly impacts facial symmetry. This habit can lead to a recessed chin, less defined jawline, and generally weaker facial structure. Mouth breathers often face abnormal jaw alignment, narrower dental arches, and an increased risk of airway obstruction. Similarly, poor posture contributes to asymmetry by creating uneven tension in facial muscles and bones. Habitual slouching or head tilting can cause imbalances in the muscles supporting the jaw and neck, consequently misaligning the temporomandibular joint (TMJ) and leading to asymmetrical muscle growth. Furthermore, bad posture can also lead to spinal misalignments that impair nerve activity and blood supply to the face, accordingly exacerbating facial asymmetry.

As already mentioned, nutrient deficiencies do not just affect our health on a microscopic level; they sculpt our very appearance, particularly when it comes to our dental and facial development:

- **Vitamin D3 deficiency**: Imagine a building where the floors do not quite line up due to foundational issues. Similarly, a prolonged lack of vitamin D3 can lead to skeletal malocclusion, a condition where the upper and lower jaws are misaligned. This misalignment affects how the teeth fit together and can skew facial symmetry much like a lopsided structure.
- **Acute malnutrition**: Inadequate protein or energy intake can impair the development of facial muscles and lead to the loss of buccal fat pads, which give

cheeks their fullness. This can leave the face looking hollow and asymmetrical.

- **Delayed tooth development and eruption**: Think of teeth as players in an orchestra each needing to arrive on cue. Nutritional deficiencies, like those causing vitamin D-resistant rickets, delay these arrivals. This mistiming disrupts the jaw's alignment and teeth arrangement, subsequently throwing off the facial harmony and balance in due course.

ESSENTIAL NUTRIENTS FOR A WINNING SMILE

Focusing on specific vitamins, nutrients, and minerals crucial for the development of facial bones and muscles is vital for promoting optimal facial growth and symmetry. Several nutrients play key roles in supporting bone density, muscle function, and overall facial structure.

Calcium: The Architect of Facial Structure

Calcium is a critical mineral essential for maintaining the strength and density of bones throughout the body, including facial bones. It serves as a foundational component in bone structure providing the necessary support for skeletal integrity. It acts much like the steel framework in skyscrapers providing the strength that keeps buildings upright under stress.

Specifically focusing on facial bones, calcium plays a pivotal role in their development and maintenance. Adequate calcium intake is crucial during periods of rapid growth, such as childhood and adolescence, to support the formation of facial bones and ensure proper facial symmetry. Without sufficient calcium, the bones may become weak and prone to deformities impacting not only facial appearance but also overall skeletal health.

Calcium is commonly obtained from dairy products, such as milk, cheese, and yogurt, which offer easily absorbed forms of the mineral. Also, plant-based calcium is available in leafy green vegetables like broccoli, spinach, and kale making them a good option for those with dietary preferences or constraints. Plus, foods that have been fortified with calcium, such as juices, plant-based milk substitutes, and specific cereals, can assist people in achieving their daily needs. Ensuring a consistent intake of calcium-rich foods is like keeping the construction of a building on schedule and up to code.

Vitamin D: The Gatekeeper of Calcium

The health and development of bones, including facial and jaw bones, depends on vitamin D because it improves the absorption of calcium. It is akin to a foreman on a construction site directing calcium to the right places to ensure proper bone growth and maintenance. Without sufficient vitamin D, even with ample calcium intake, the body struggles to maintain bone density.

Vitamin D is essential for the mineralization and remodeling of bone tissue and maintaining the structural integrity of the jaw and other facial bones. This is especially important during growth phases such as childhood and adolescence when facial bones are actively forming and developing.

The body synthesizes vitamin D primarily through exposure to sunlight. But during winter months or in northern latitudes, fortified foods and supplements become crucial to prevent deficiencies. Additionally, it can be obtained from dietary sources like eggs, fortified foods such as milk, orange juice, and cereal, as well as fatty fish like tuna and salmon. To ensure adequate levels of this vital nutrient, it is important to spend some time in the sunlight and include these vitamin D-rich foods in your diet to keep this gatekeeper alert.

Phosphorus: Calcium's Partner in Crime

Phosphorus teams up with calcium working behind the scenes to fortify the strength and structure of your teeth and facial bones. This partnership is crucial for the maintenance and repair of all body tissues, but phosphorus is super important for keeping your teeth healthy too. It helps make and take care of the hard outer layer of your teeth, which keeps them safe from decay and harm.

Phosphorus is found in foods like meat, fish, dairy, nuts, seeds, and beans. Eating these foods helps your body get enough phosphorus, which is important for keeping your bones strong and helping jaw and facial bones grow properly.

Vitamin A: The Protector of Your Smile

Vitamin A plays a pivotal role in oral health as the secret weapon for developing strong, decay-resistant tooth enamel. Adequate vitamin A ensures that enamel—the hard, protective outer layer of your teeth—is properly formed, hence safeguarding your smile against cavities and erosion. Beyond just defending your teeth, vitamin A is also a guardian for your overall facial aesthetics.

This vitamin is crucial in maintaining the health of mucous membranes and skin—fundamental components that define your face's structure and appearance. It promotes the repair and growth of bodily tissues, especially within the gums and the inner linings of the cheeks, accordingly enhancing the body's ability to naturally cleanse the mouth and reduce the risk of infections. Furthermore, vitamin A boosts saliva production, which is essential for washing away bacteria and maintaining oral hygiene. It also supports skin health by regulating and stimulating sebum and collagen production that keeps the skin resilient and prevents premature aging, respectively.

Rich in vitamin A, foods like liver and dairy products such as cheese and milk are potent dental health allies. For those preferring plant-based sources, carrots, sweet potatoes, and leafy greens like spinach and kale are invaluable. These foods contain beta-carotene, which the body converts into vitamin A, ultimately helping to fortify your defenses against oral health issues and keep your smile radiant and healthy.

Vitamin C: The Sculptor of Collagen

Vitamin C is an essential nutrient that is vital for maintaining oral health, particularly in promoting gum health. It aids in preserving the integrity of the gums by protecting against gum disease and the risk of tooth loss. The role of vitamin C in collagen production is crucial, as it helps keep the gums robust and resilient, therefore effectively supporting the teeth and preventing the breakdown of gum tissues. This nutrient also possesses anti-inflammatory properties, which protect against conditions like gingivitis by reducing swelling and bleeding in the gums.

Dietary sources of vitamin C are abundant and include citrus fruits like oranges and lemons, strawberries, bell peppers, and broccoli. These foods not only boost levels of this essential nutrient but also provide a variety of other beneficial compounds that support overall health. Incorporating these vitamin C-rich foods into your diet can help ensure optimal skin health and contribute to maintaining a robust immune system, which together lay the foundation for a glowing, well-protected facial appearance.

Protein: The Muscle Builder

Protein is the building block of the body essential not just for building muscle but also for enhancing facial aesthetics and functionality. It plays a vital role in strengthening the muscles responsible for expressions and chewing, thereby ensuring facial symmetry and expressiveness. The amino acids in protein are critical for the synthesis and repair of muscle fibers and other tissues in the face, thus aiding in recovery and maintaining the health and vibrancy of your appearance.

Incorporating high-protein foods into your diet is key to these benefits. Lean meats such as turkey, chicken, and specific cuts of beef like sirloin and tenderloin provide high-quality protein without excess fat. Fish, eggs, beans, lentils, and tofu also offer rich sources of protein. Regular consumption of these foods ensures that your facial muscles are well-maintained for optimal strength and functionality, supports overall facial symmetry, and contributes to a healthier, more attractive appearance.

Magnesium: The Enhancer

Magnesium is an essential element that enhances the effectiveness of calcium and vitamin D to support the formation of healthy bones, including the structural integrity of the bones in the jaw and face. Magnesium helps with calcium absorption and usage, which guarantees that it is correctly incorporated into bone tissue, while calcium offers the foundation for strong bones. Magnesium significantly strengthens vitamin D's involvement in bone health by aiding in its activation.

Specifically focusing on the jaw and facial bones, magnesium contributes to the mineralization process, therefore helping to build and maintain strong and resilient bone structure. Adequate magnesium intake is essential for ensuring the proper formation and density of facial bones, which are integral for facial symmetry and overall skeletal integrity.

Foods such as brown rice and quinoa, nuts such as cashews and almonds, and leafy green vegetables like kale and spinach are rich dietary sources of magnesium.

Omega-3 Fatty Acids: The Inflammation Fighter

Omega-3 fatty acids are celebrated for their remarkable benefits for the skin and facial muscles by playing a key role in enhancing overall health and appearance. Their powerful anti-inflammatory properties help soothe inflammation in both skin and muscles, eventually fostering a vibrant complexion and efficient muscle function. By maintaining moisture and enhancing elasticity, omega-3s combat dryness and prevent the signs of aging such as wrinkles, contributing to a youthful and healthy skin texture as a result.

Additionally, omega-3 fatty acids are instrumental in managing skin conditions like acne, eczema, and psoriasis, promoting healing, and maintaining smooth, clear skin. They also support the health of facial muscles by aiding in their repair and recovery, which is crucial for maintaining facial symmetry, tone, and definition. This contributes to an overall enhanced appearance and vitality. To reap these benefits, include omega-3 rich foods in your diet such as salmon, mackerel, sardines, flaxseeds, chia seeds, and walnuts, which provide a robust foundation for both skin health and muscle functionality.

Zinc: The Unsung Hero

Zinc, often hailed as the "unsung hero" of nutrients, plays a pivotal role in maintaining a healthy smile. This essential mineral is crucial for numerous biological functions, including aiding in plaque and tartar control on teeth and supporting the healing of gum tissues. Zinc's antibacterial properties help reduce the growth of bacteria that can cause bad breath and gum disease. Moreover, it is integral to wound healing and tissue repair—processes vital for recovering from dental procedures and maintaining overall oral health. By boosting the immune system, zinc also helps the body fight off oral infections more effectively, safeguarding the health of your gums and teeth later on.

A variety of foods offer rich sources of zinc, thereby ensuring that both meat-eaters and vegetarians can benefit. Meats, particularly beef and poultry, are excellent sources of highly bioavailable zinc, which means the zinc they contain is readily absorbed by the body. Shellfish, such as oysters, crab, and shrimp, are not only rich in zinc but also add a gourmet touch to diets. For those who prefer plant-based sources, legumes like beans, lentils, and chickpeas provide a substantial amount of zinc making it easy to incorporate this unsung hero into your diet to support a robust, healthy smile.

Fiber: The Cleanser

Fiber is crucial for oral health, as it helps maintain a clean and healthy mouth. High-fiber foods stimulate saliva flow—the mouth's natural cleanser. This increased saliva production helps rinse away food particles and neutralize harmful acids that attack tooth enamel, hence significantly reducing the risk of cavities and gum disease. Furthermore, the act of chewing fibrous foods like apples and carrots provides a natural scrubbing action on the teeth and helps to keep them clean. Fiber's role in promoting digestive health also contributes to better oral health indirectly, as a healthy digestive system can reduce the prevalence of mouth bacteria.

Sources of fiber-rich foods are abundant, ensuring that everyone can incorporate more fiber into their diets. Apples and carrots, for instance, are not only packed with nutrients but also have a high fiber content that helps clean teeth while eating them. Leafy greens like spinach and kale are excellent sources of fiber and provide a multitude of other vitamins and minerals beneficial for gum health. Whole grains and legumes, including beans and lentils, also contribute significant amounts of fiber to the diet. By including these foods regularly, you ensure an effective natural cleaning process in your oral care regimen, ultimately enhancing your overall dental hygiene and health.

Water: The Essential Life Force

Water is essential to life, as it fulfills crucial functions within the body such as nutrient transport, body temperature regulation, and toxin removal. Staying hydrated keeps the skin supple and vibrant, helping to minimize wrinkles and maintain a youthful complexion. It is also vital for producing saliva.

Moreover, water plays a key role in oral and facial health. Adequate hydration ensures that the muscles and bones of the face remain healthy, thus facilitating optimum muscle function and preventing cramps or fatigue. Regular water intake is vital not only for keeping facial structures robust but also for supporting overall bodily health making it indispensable for a healthy smile and a vibrant appearance.

CRUNCH TIME

In Chapter 1, the link between food and facial structure emphasizes how our diet shapes our facial features. Historically, diets comprised tougher, fibrous foods requiring significant chewing, therefore stimulating jawbone growth and yielding wider jaws with aligned teeth. But modern diets dominated by processed, soft foods reduce the need for vigorous chewing and lead to underdeveloped jaws and dental misalignments. This trend often results in overcrowded teeth and impacts breathing and facial aesthetics.

Chewing Crunchy Foods Help Your Jaw and Teeth.

Chewing crunchy foods provides a natural workout for your jaw muscles and maintains the strength and integrity of your teeth. When you consume crunchy foods like apples, carrots, or nuts, the act of chewing requires more effort compared to softer foods. This increased effort stimulates blood flow to the gums and jawbone and promotes overall oral health. Also, eating crunchy foods with a rough texture can help clean your teeth by scraping away plaque and leftover food bits. This natural cleansing action can improve your oral hygiene. Regularly chewing crunchy foods can also maintain proper jaw alignment and reduce the risk of TMJ disorders by strengthening the jaw-supporting muscles.

Importance of Crunchy Foods

Incorporating crunchy foods into your diet offers multiple benefits ranging from enhancing digestion to improving oral and facial health. High in fiber, crunchy foods like apples and raw vegetables not only satisfy hunger effectively but also help manage weight by preventing overeating. Soluble fiber from these foods nourishes gut bacteria and facilitates regular bowel movements, while the insoluble type adds bulk to help prevent constipation.

Chewing crunchy foods also serves as a natural workout that strengthens and tones your facial and jaw muscles. This action not only promotes better chewing efficiency and speech articulation but also triggers the production of saliva, which cleanses the teeth and remineralizes enamel to reduce the risk of decay. Moreover, the repetitive chewing of hard textures stimulates collagen production—essential for maintaining skin elasticity and firmness. This can help prevent skin sagging and the formation of wrinkles contributing to a youthful appearance and improved facial symmetry. Including a variety of crunchy foods in your meals not only diversifies your diet but also enhances sensory satisfaction with vibrant textures and flavors, elevating the overall dining experience in due course.

When considering good crunchy vegetables for children, it is important to focus on options that not only provide a satisfying crunch but also offer valuable nutrients and fiber. Here are examples falling under each category.

Crunchy, fibrous vegetables

- **Carrots:** Crunchy and naturally sweet, carrots are a hit with kids and a great source of beta-carotene—vital for maintaining good eyesight. Perfect for on-the-go snacking, carrot sticks or baby carrots offer a convenient boost of nutrition.

- **Celery:** Known for its satisfying crunch, celery pairs wonderfully with dips like peanut butter or hummus. It is a low-calorie option rich in fiber, hence supporting digestive wellness with every crisp bite.
- **Bell peppers:** These vibrant vegetables add a pop of color and crunch to any meal. Available in red, green, and yellow, bell peppers are not only visually appealing but also rich in vitamin C—essential for a robust immune system. They are perfect when sliced into salads or served with dip for a nutritious snack.
- **Snap peas:** Crisp and a sweet flavor, snap peas are a favorite among children. Rich in fiber and vitamin K, they support bone health and can be enjoyed raw or lightly steamed making them a versatile and healthy choice.
- **Cucumber:** Cucumbers have a refreshing crunch and a high water content i.e., hydrating abilities. They are low in calories and can be sliced into rounds or sticks for easy snacking.

Crunchy, fibrous fruits

- **Apples:** Apples, beloved by many children for their crunchy texture, are rich in fiber and vitamin C.
- **Pears:** Pears have a crunchy texture when ripe and are sweet and juicy. They contain dietary fiber, which aids digestion. Sliced pears can be served with cheese or yogurt for a balanced snack.

- **Grapes:** Providing a delightful crunch and packed with antioxidants and vitamin C, grapes are not only easy to eat but also versatile; you can enjoy them fresh or frozen for a refreshing treat on a warm day. Their convenience and nutritional benefits make grapes an excellent choice for healthy snacking.
- **Kiwi:** Kiwi has a unique combination of crunchiness from its seeds and softness from its flesh. It is loaded with vitamin C and dietary fiber. Kiwi slices can be added to fruit salads or enjoyed on their own.
- **Pineapple:** Pineapple brings a taste of the tropics with its sweet flavor and fibrous, crunchy texture. It is an excellent source of vitamin C and manganese, essential for antioxidant defense and energy production. Fresh pineapple chunks are perfect for snacking by adding a burst of flavor and nutrition to your day.

QUICK RECAP

- **Balanced diet:** Essential for oral and airway health, it provides vital nutrients for development and maintenance.
- **Teeth health:** Calcium, phosphorus, and vitamin D are crucial for strong teeth and enamel formation.
- **Gum health:** Vitamin C is necessary for gum integrity and collagen production.
- **Facial structure:** Proper nutrition supports jaw development and airway function.

- **Prevention of oral diseases:** Balanced diet is crucial for avoiding tooth decay and gum disease.
- **Impact of modern diets:** Processed foods can hinder proper palate formation leading to dental and respiratory issues.
- **Early intervention:** Promoting healthy eating habits in childhood reduces the risk of respiratory problems and supports overall well-being.

In the upcoming chapter, we will discuss the connection between sleep quality and respiratory health, learn to identify sleep-related breathing conditions, and create a conducive sleep environment for quality sleep i.e., better respiratory health.

CHAPTER 7
SWEET DREAMS ARE MADE OF THESE

While it may initially seem endearing to hear your child snoring—reminiscent of family traits—it is essential not to dismiss it lightly. Snoring in children can be a significant indicator of a deeper issue, such as OSA where breathing difficulties arise during sleep. This condition can lead to several challenges for children, which include hyperactivity, difficulty concentrating, and emotional and social struggles. Unfortunately, these symptoms often get misinterpreted as ADHD. This results in the administration of medications that may worsen the underlying sleep problem rather than addressing it. With approximately 2.4 million children in the U.S. diagnosed with ADHD, it is important to consider that what appears to be ADHD may actually stem from untreated sleep disorders.

Observing your child's sleep patterns and identifying signs such as snoring, fatigue, dark circles under the eyes, bedwetting, nightmares, morning headaches, or enlarged tonsils and adenoids is paramount. These signs and symptoms could suggest OSA rather than ADHD. Before settling on an ADHD diagnosis, it is imperative to engage in discussions with your child's pediatrician or dentist regarding these symptoms. Such could lead to a reassessment of the situation and potentially alter the course of treatment, significantly impacting the quality of life for your child later on.

THE BREATH OF NIGHT

Quality sleep is essential for optimal respiratory health by playing a critical role in maintaining lung function and overall well-being. During sleep, the respiratory system experiences vital physiological changes that help clear airways, regulate breathing patterns, and ensure efficient oxygen exchange. This restorative process is crucial not only for the body but also for mental clarity and function.

Sleep impacts various bodily systems, particularly the lungs. Although the full purpose of sleep is not entirely understood, it is clear that it does more than just provide rest—it enhances several physiological functions including respiratory ones. Conversely, a lack of sleep can have negative effects on the body. Sleep deprivation increases stress levels leading to rapid breathing and potentially complicating conditions for those with existing respiratory issues. Thus, ensuring sufficient sleep is crucial for supporting the respiratory system and maintaining overall health.

Effects of Lack of Sleep to Your Respiratory System

Getting insufficient sleep not only leaves you feeling tired but also negatively impacts your respiratory system. Poor sleep weakens your immune system, thus increasing susceptibility to respiratory illnesses. For individuals with chronic lung conditions such as asthma or COPD, lack of sleep can worsen symptoms and make breathing more challenging. Additionally, inadequate sleep is linked to a higher risk of serious health issues including depression, diabetes, kidney disease, and stroke, hence highlighting the essential role of adequate sleep in overall health.

Sleep disturbances also directly affect breathing patterns. During sleep, brain activity slows leading to variations in breathing depth and regularity, which are particularly evident as we cycle between non-rapid eye movement (NREM) and rapid eye movement (REM) sleep. In REM sleep where dreams are most vivid and muscle activity is reduced, breathing can become shallower and less frequent, thus complicating respiratory processes. Furthermore, respiratory conditions, smoking, or physical obstructions can disrupt sleep by obstructing the body to adequately oxygenate the blood. This disturbance in normal sleep patterns exacerbates respiratory issues and perpetuates sleep disruptions, hence underscoring the interconnectedness of sleep quality and respiratory health.

Changes in Breathing Patterns During Different Sleep Stages

Understanding these sleep stages helps you grasp how your sleep quality impacts your health. Sleep usually goes through different stages starting from light sleep, going deeper, and then into rapid eye movement (REM) sleep. This cycle repeats multiple times during a regular night's sleep:

1. **Stage 1—light sleep:** This is when you are simply falling off and can be quickly awakened. It is a brief period usually lasting several minutes during which muscle activity decreases and you may experience unexpected muscle contractions or a sensation of falling.

2. **Stage 2—onset of sleep:** During this stage, your body begins to relax more deeply. Your heart rate and breathing rate slow down, and your body temperature decreases. This stage accounts for a significant portion of total sleep time in adults.

3. **Stage 3—restorative deep sleep:** During this phase of sleep, the body undergoes significant restoration by repairing tissues, generating bone and muscle, and enhancing the immune system. Waking someone during this stage can be challenging, and they may feel disoriented for a brief period upon awakening. Deep sleep is particularly beneficial for children and adolescents.

4. **REM sleep:** This stage starts about 90 min after going to sleep and lasts for many hours during the night with each subsequent REM stage lasting longer

than the previous one. Faster breathing and heart rate, heightened brain activity, rapid eye movements, and momentary paralysis of the arm and leg muscles are all signs of REM sleep. The majority of dreams happen during REM sleep, which is crucial for processing stress, memories, and emotions.

The sleep cycle is dynamic i.e., changing in duration throughout the night. Early in the night, restorative deep sleep predominates and makes up a large portion of the sleep cycle. As the night progresses, REM sleep stages extend, particularly in the latter half. Each sleep cycle lasts about 90–110 min with adults typically experiencing 4–6 cycles each night. Insufficient cycles or disruptions in the sleep cycle can lead to fragmented sleep, which diminishes the restorative benefits of sleep and leaves individuals feeling unrefreshed. For those with respiratory issues, disrupted or inadequate sleep can lead to fatigue, reduced disease resistance, and worsened respiratory function over time.

RECOGNIZING SLEEP ISSUES

Airway health-related sleep disorders can affect both adults and children, but knowledge about these problems can diminish fears and encourage preventative care. The following are the common sleep issues related to airway health along with their symptoms, risks, and potential effects on general health.

Obstructive Sleep Apnea

OSA is a syndrome characterized by breathing disruptions during sleep caused by the relaxation of neck muscles, which leads to airway obstruction. This causes recurrent breathing pauses when the airway narrows or collapses, preventing oxygen from reaching the lungs in consequence. While these breathing disruptions are often brief, they occur frequently throughout the night, hence disturbing the usual sleep cycle.

Loud snoring is one of the most noticeable signs of OSA. Along with snoring, OSA sufferers frequently have disturbed sleep due to regular disruption of their sleep by bouts of choking or gasping for air as the body tries to regain normal breathing.

OSA patients frequently experience daytime fatigue. Despite spending what appears to be a fair amount of time in bed, people with OSA wake up feeling unrefreshed and lethargic throughout the day. Persistent weariness can have serious consequences for daily functioning including focus, productivity, and mood disruption. Significant dangers to general health such as cardiovascular problems and daytime fatigue are associated with OSA, which negatively impacts daily functioning and quality of life.

Snoring

Snoring, while often dismissed as a minor annoyance, may actually be a key OSA indicator. Contrary to the myth that snoring is a sign of deep sleep, it actually signifies potential airway obstruction and poor sleep quality. Particularly in children with enlarged tonsils or adenoids, snoring and other symptoms like bedwetting, poor growth, and concentration difficulties in school may suggest OSA.

The idea that snoring equates to deep sleep is a persistent myth. Actually, snoring can cause fragmented and restless sleep patterns by interfering with its quality. Recognizing the potential seriousness of snoring is crucial, especially when accompanied by other symptoms such as daytime fatigue or witnessed breathing pauses during sleep. Such signs may warrant further evaluation for sleep apnea to prevent potential complications.

You should note that not everyone who snores has sleep apnea. Anatomical differences in the airway or obesity and alcohol consumption are common causes of snoring. Changing one's lifestyle to include things like losing weight, abstaining from alcohol before bed, and sleeping on one's side will frequently reduce snoring. In addition, snoring caused by sleep apnea can be efficiently managed with medical measures, such as continuous positive airway pressure (CPAP) therapy and oral appliances.

Nocturnal Asthma

Nocturnal asthma presents a unique challenge for asthma sufferers, as it refers to asthma symptoms that appear during sleep such as coughing, wheezing, or difficulty breathing. Unlike daytime asthma symptoms, which can be induced by environmental causes such as allergens or exercise, nocturnal asthma worsens at night, alters sleep patterns, and negatively impacts your health.

Various factors can contribute to nocturnal asthma, including allergens like dust mites or pet dander, exposure to irritants such as tobacco smoke or strong odors, changes in temperature or humidity levels, and even hormonal fluctuations.

Proper asthma management plays a key role in alleviating symptoms and improving sleep quality for individuals with nocturnal asthma. This includes adherence to prescribed asthma medications, such as inhalers or oral medications, as well as understanding how and when to use them to effectively control symptoms. Long-term control medications, like inhaled corticosteroids or leukotriene modifiers, can help reduce airway inflammation and prevent asthma flare-ups including those that occur during sleep.

In addition to medication management, avoiding triggers is critical to reducing nocturnal asthma symptoms. This could include making modifications to the sleep environment such as utilizing hypoallergenic bedding, vacuuming and dusting on a regular basis to limit allergy exposure, and keeping the bedroom at a consistent temperature and humidity level. It is also critical to detect and treat any concomitant illnesses that may contribute to nocturnal asthma, such as gastroesophageal reflux disease (GERD) or OSA.

Allergic Rhinitis

Allergic rhinitis, colloquially known as hay fever, emerges as a common allergic response triggered by environmental allergens. When exposed to substances like pollen, dust mites, pet dander, or mold spores, susceptible individuals mount an immune reaction characterized by inflammation of the nasal passages. This inflammation manifests through a range of symptoms including persistent sneezing, nasal congestion, and a runny or itchy nose.

The effects of allergic rhinitis go beyond discomfort throughout the day and interfere with sleep. When nasal congestion worsens at night, it obstructs the airway and makes it difficult for air to pass through. This blockage has the potential to induce or worsen episodes of snoring and disrupt the normal circadian rhythm. Not only can these conditions cause sleep disturbances but also trigger other issues like fatigue, irritability, and diminished cognitive function during waking hours.

To mitigate the effects of allergic rhinitis, reducing allergen exposure and employing appropriate medical treatments are essential. Customize your environment to limit contact with allergens by identifying specific triggers through allergy testing. Consider using allergen-proof bedding, installing air purifiers, and limiting outdoor activities during high pollen seasons to further protect against allergic reactions.

Also, medical treatment options offer valuable relief from allergic rhinitis symptoms. Over-the-counter antihistamines and decongestants can help alleviate nasal congestion and sneezing, while nasal corticosteroids effectively target inflammation within the nasal passages. In cases of severe or persistent symptoms, allergen immunotherapy administered through allergy shots or sublingual tablets may be recommended to desensitize the immune system to specific allergens over time.

Tonsil Troubles

Enlarged tonsils and adenoids can severely affect a child's breathing, particularly during sleep, and may lead to sleep disorders such as OSA. Located at the back of the throat and in the nasal cavity, tonsils and adenoids are crucial parts of the immune system. However, when they become enlarged, they can block the airway and cause breathing issues at night.

A recurring indication that a child might need tonsil or adenoid removal is frequent throat infections. Enlarged tonsils can harbor bacteria resulting in repeated cases of tonsillitis or sore throats. Additionally, enlarged tonsils can hinder the passage of food and fluids leading to difficulty swallowing (dysphagia), which causes discomfort or pain. This can be particularly distressing for parents and may impact a child's nutrition and hydration.

Persistent snoring or breathing difficulties during sleep are clear indicators that enlarged tonsils or adenoids may be obstructing the airway. Such obstructions can lead to OSA when breathing repeatedly stops and starts during sleep. Symptoms in children may include breathing pauses, gasping for air, or restless sleep, all of which can impair sleep quality, cause daytime tiredness, and lead to behavioral problems.

When enlarged tonsils or adenoids significantly obstruct the airway, surgical removal through a tonsillectomy or adenoidectomy is often recommended. This common procedure is performed under general anesthesia. By removing the obstructive tissues, the airway is opened up, which improves airflow during sleep, alleviates symptoms of

OSA, reduces the frequency of throat infections, and enhances overall sleep quality and daytime alertness.

Parents should vigilantly watch for symptoms of airway obstruction in their child such as repeated infections, difficulty swallowing, and sleep-related breathing problems. Nonetheless, any decision to proceed with surgery should involve close consultation with a healthcare professional. Prompt medical intervention not only alleviates these troubling symptoms but also prevents the long-term health complications associated with enlarged tonsils or adenoids, thereby safeguarding your child's future well-being.

A DREAMY SLEEP ENVIRONMENT

Creating a sleep-conducive environment is essential for promoting better sleep quality and respiratory health. The following tips will help you achieve this.

Maintain a Cool, Comfortable Temperature

To promote respiratory health and facilitate restful sleep, it is crucial to maintain a cool and comfortable temperature in the bedroom. Ideally, the temperature should be set between 65–70 °F to foster an environment conducive to peaceful sleep.

Overly warm bedroom temperatures can hinder the body's ability to regulate its own temperature leading to discomfort and difficulties falling asleep. High temperatures can cause excessive sweating that disrupts sleep and may worsen respiratory issues, particularly in individuals with asthma or allergies. Moreover, warmer conditions can lead to dehydration that negatively impacts both overall health and respiratory function.

Excessively cold temperatures can also detract from sleep quality. When the body is too cold, it struggles to maintain a state conducive to restful, restorative sleep. Moreover, cold air can irritate the respiratory system causing airway inflammation and aggravating symptoms in those with respiratory conditions.

Extreme temperatures—whether too hot or too cold—can disrupt the body's natural sleep-wake cycle leading to poor sleep and reduced overall sleep quality. This disruption affects not just physical health but also cognitive function, mood, and immune response. Ensuring that your bedroom maintains a comfortable temperature is essential for good sleep and respiratory health by helping the body to relax properly and reduce the risk of breathing difficulties. A well-regulated sleeping environment is key to enhancing overall well-being.

Ensure Proper Ventilation

Having proper ventilation is crucial for keeping indoor environments healthy because it guarantees enough airflow. There are several reasons why good ventilation is important ranging from health considerations to environmental factors.

First and foremost, ventilation lessens the possibility of backdrafting, which happens when exhaust gasses—like carbon monoxide—are sucked back into the house as opposed to being released outside. Because backdrafting can result in carbon monoxide poisoning—a potentially fatal condition—it poses major health risks. Ventilation systems aid in preventing the accumulation of dangerous gasses and preserving a safe living environment by encouraging adequate airflow.

Good ventilation is crucial for maintaining respiratory health and managing conditions like asthma, as it helps clear indoor air of pollutants like dust, mold spores, and volatile organic compounds (VOCs). These contaminants, often released from household products such as paints, cleaning agents, and furniture, can accumulate indoors due to poor ventilation, therefore exacerbating allergies and asthma symptoms. Effective ventilation not only improves indoor air quality but also filters out allergens like pollen and pet dander, subsequently reducing the likelihood of allergic reactions and respiratory distress for individuals with sensitivities.

By promoting the dispersal of VOCs and other airborne irritants, proper ventilation systems create a healthier living environment. This is especially important, as prolonged exposure to high levels of VOCs can lead to respiratory irritation and neurological symptoms. That being so, ensuring robust ventilation contributes significantly to reducing the concentration of these compounds indoors and minimizes various health risks, enhancing overall well-being as a result.

Ventilation systems also play a crucial role in reducing radon gas levels—a radioactive gas that seeps into homes from the soil. Radon exposure is a major health concern, as it is the second leading cause of lung cancer after smoking. Effective ventilation promotes air exchange that helps dilute radon concentrations, thereby mitigating the risk of exposure and protecting respiratory health.

Use Hypoallergenic Bedding

Opting for hypoallergenic bedding is key for those looking to minimize their exposure to allergens such as dust mites, mold, and pet dander, which can worsen respiratory issues during sleep. Among the various materials, silk is particularly notable for its luxurious feel and natural hypoallergenic qualities. It resists dust mites and mold, consequently providing a clean, allergen-free sleep surface while its smooth texture soothes sensitive skin. Bamboo is another excellent choice prized for its sustainability and breathability along with antimicrobial properties that deter allergens and help maintain a cool, dry bed environment. For the colder months, wool is favored for its natural insulation and ability to resist dust mites and mold. Linen—durable and breathable—also offers hypoallergenic properties and resistance to dust mites, thus ensuring a dry and comfortable sleeping environment that helps reduce allergen buildup.

Control Humidity Levels

Maintaining the right level of humidity in your bedroom is crucial for comfortable and healthy sleep. Humidity, which measures the amount of water vapor in the air, plays a vital role in how well you breathe and your overall comfort. When the air is too dry, it can lead to a variety of respiratory issues including a dry throat, irritated nasal passages, and an increased likelihood of respiratory infections. Dry air can aggravate symptoms of conditions like asthma and allergies by causing airway irritation and inflammation. Introducing a humidifier to your bedroom can help alleviate these issues by adding necessary moisture to the air, enhancing your breathing comfort, and facilitating better sleep.

On the flip side, excessively high humidity levels can also negatively impact respiratory health. In such humid environments, the air's characteristics compound respiratory challenges. High humidity levels encourage the growth of mold, dust mites, and other allergens, which can exacerbate breathing difficulties, particularly for individuals with asthma and allergies. Employing a dehumidifier to reduce moisture levels can significantly improve air quality in your home, aid in the prevention of respiratory issues, and create a healthier sleeping environment.

Maintaining a balanced humidity level in the bedroom is essential for optimal sleep quality and respiratory health. It is crucial to regularly check humidity levels, particularly during seasons or in climates with significant humidity changes. Using a hygrometer—a device that measures humidity—can help you decide if you need a humidifier or dehumidifier to achieve the ideal conditions for a comfortable and healthful sleep environment.

Minimize Allergens and Irritants

Minimizing allergens and irritants in the bedroom is crucial for promoting better respiratory health and ensuring a restful night's sleep. This involves a comprehensive approach aimed at reducing the presence of common triggers such as dust mites, pet dander, and airborne particles. Nonetheless, you can follow the next tips.

Regular cleaning, dusting, and vacuuming are fundamental steps in allergen control. Dusting surfaces (furniture, shelves, and baseboards) removes accumulated dust and prevents its redistribution into the air. Vacuuming with a high efficiency particulate air (HEPA) filter-equipped vacuum cleaner effectively captures dust and allergens from carpets, rugs, and upholstery preventing them from being stirred up and inhaled.

Removing or limiting possible reservoirs for dust mites and other allergens like plush toys, heavy drapes, and decorative pillows reduces the overall dust load in the bedroom, as these contribute to respiratory irritation and allergy symptoms.

Washing your bedding, pillows without covers, and stuffed toys every week in hot water (at least 130 °F) kills dust mites and gets rid of allergens. Using a hot dryer cycle further ensures the elimination of dust mites, as they cannot survive high temperatures. This regular washing routine is essential for maintaining a clean sleeping environment and minimizing exposure to allergens that can disrupt sleep and exacerbate respiratory conditions.

It is important to prevent pet dander buildup in bedrooms, especially for people allergic to pets. You can do this by keeping pets out of the bedroom, grooming them often to reduce shedding, and using air purifiers with HEPA filters to trap pet dander in the air.

Provide Comfortable Sleepwear

Choosing comfortable sleepwear is important for getting good sleep and keeping your breathing healthy. It is not just about the bed and blankets; the clothes you wear to bed matter too.

First and foremost, selecting breathable and comfortable pajamas is key. Breathability ensures proper airflow around the body that prevents overheating and excessive sweating during sleep. Natural fabrics like cotton, linen, and bamboo are great for sleeping because they let air move around easily to keep you cool and comfy all night. These fabrics also absorb moisture, accordingly maintaining optimal skin conditions and reducing the risk of skin irritation.

On the other hand, artificial fabrics like fleece can hold onto heat and sweat close to your skin, making you feel uncomfortable and causing sleep problems as a result. These materials lack breathability and can contribute to overheating, especially in warmer climates or during periods of heightened physical activity. By avoiding synthetic fabrics, individuals can mitigate the risk of excessive sweating and discomfort, thereby promoting better sleep quality and respiratory health.

It is important to avoid tight or restrictive sleepwear, as it can hinder circulation and breathing. Tight clothing may constrict blood flow, subsequently causing discomfort, numbness, and tingling. Restrictive garments can also limit the movement of the chest and abdomen, thus impeding deep breathing during sleep. Opting for loose-fitting pajamas allows for unrestricted movement and better airflow around the body, which improves comfort and promotes relaxed breathing.

Consider Sleep Position

The sleep position is important in managing various respiratory issues by either facilitating or impeding airflow during sleep. Elevating the head slightly can be particularly beneficial for individuals struggling with congestion or breathing difficulties. By positioning the head higher than the rest of the body, gravity helps to drain nasal passages, hence reducing congestion and promoting easier breathing. This slight elevation can also alleviate symptoms associated with conditions like sinusitis or allergies, by and by allowing for a more restful night's sleep.

For those who snore, sleep position is crucial. Sleeping on the back can cause the tongue and throat tissues to fall back, partially blocking the airway and leading to snoring and potential sleep apnea episodes. Switching to sleeping on one's side can help keep the airway open and prevent the soft tissues from collapsing. By avoiding the supine position where the back is flat against the mattress, individuals can reduce the likelihood of snoring and enhance sleep quality.

QUICK RECAP

- Snoring in children can indicate deeper health issues like OSA, often misdiagnosed as ADHD.
- Pay attention to signs like snoring, fatigue, bedwetting, and enlarged tonsils for potential sleep disorders.
- Awareness of the four sleep stages (NREM 1, NREM

2, NREM 3, REM) aids in understanding sleep patterns and their impact on respiratory health.

- Lack of quality sleep affects the respiratory system, weakens immunity, exacerbates chronic lung conditions, and increases the risk of serious health issues.
- Common sleep issues like OSA, snoring, nocturnal asthma, allergic rhinitis, and tonsil troubles affect respiratory health and require proactive management.
- Tips include maintaining temperature and humidity levels, proper ventilation, using hypoallergenic bedding, minimizing allergens, and considering comfortable sleepwear and positions.
- Treatment options for sleep disorders vary and may involve lifestyle adjustments, medical interventions like CPAP therapy, or surgical procedures.

The next chapter will discuss the role of orthodontics in airway development. You will gain insights into how timely orthodontic interventions can positively impact airway health in children.

CHAPTER 8
STRAIGHT TALK

Healthy teeth have always been valued for their function and appearance—a fact emphasized by ancient practices of dental correction. Many ancient civilizations used a crude form of braces not only to straighten crowded teeth among the living but also ensure that the deceased had perfectly aligned smiles for their journey into the afterlife.

The ancient Egyptians cleverly attached metal posts to their teeth with cords made from animal intestines, similar to today's archwires, and they can even be seen on preserved mummies. The Romans, true pioneers of orthodontics, used fine gold wires as ligatures to adjust teeth in the living. These historical practices reveal how our quest for perfect smiles spans centuries, hence underscoring our enduring fascination with dental health. For today's parents, this rich history emphasizes the importance of consulting with dental professionals to ensure their children enjoy confident, radiant smiles that stand the test of time.

ORTHODONTICS: BEYOND A BEAUTIFUL SMILE

Orthodontics involves more than just aligning teeth to fit and function in a specific way; it includes enhancing breathing patterns and optimizing airway function. By techniques like arch expansion, orthodontists widen the upper or lower jawbone to promote nasal breathing and diminish mouth breathing. In fact, the roof of your mouth is like the floor of your nose. By broadening and adjusting the upper jawbone, orthodontists open up nasal passages to improve airflow. This also impacts jaw positioning, which in turn affects the tongue's placement and breathing through the throat.

Nasal breathing is crucial, as it promotes proper tongue positioning against the roof of the mouth and aids in the natural growth of the upper jaw. Conversely, mouth breathing, especially during sleep—can disrupt this process and potentially affect the formation of the upper jaw bone in children. Encouraging nasal breathing, particularly during sleep, fosters optimal jaw development and overall respiratory health.

Orthodontic treatment offers more than just cosmetic benefits; it lays the groundwork for a healthier and happier future. By addressing dental and jaw issues, you not only enhance your appearance but also improve breathing and energy levels. With orthodontic intervention, children's breathing can improve by reducing mouth breathing, which may contribute to dental irregularities if left unattended. While occasional mouth breathing is normal, persistent instances could indicate underlying concerns that an orthodontist can address, potentially averting future complications.

Orthodontic interventions play a crucial role in managing OSA. By addressing oral issues early on, orthodontists can tailor treatments to promote nasal breathing, therefore alleviating OSA symptoms like dry mouth and daytime irritability and improving sleep quality. This not only enhances physical health but also contributes to improved mental well-being for children undergoing orthodontic treatment.

How Orthodontics Improve Facial Structure

Orthodontics plays a pivotal role in improving facial structure by aligning teeth and jaws effectively. Treatments like braces or aligners gradually shift teeth into their correct positions, enhancing facial symmetry and harmony later on. By establishing a well-aligned bite and jaw relationship, orthodontics contributes to a balanced and aesthetically pleasing facial profile.

Orthodontic interventions address various dental issues including underbites where the lower teeth protrude past the upper teeth due to genetic or inherited factors. Treatment involves repositioning the lower jaw or adjusting the upper teeth to correct the misalignment.

Similarly, overbites—marked by the upper front teeth overlapping the lower ones excessively—are addressed using orthodontic methods to establish a harmonious bite. These overbites are frequently attributed to genetic factors or habits like thumb-sucking, prolonged pacifier use, or extensive bottle-feeding beyond infancy. Orthodontic intervention targets this overlap through repositioning teeth to achieve dental balance and alignment.

Additionally, orthodontics addresses malocclusion that encompasses misalignments like open bites— a gap between upper and lower front teeth even when the jaws are closed. Treatment involves realigning teeth and modifying the bite relationship to close the gap and improve overall facial aesthetics. Orthodontic evaluation and treatment are crucial for correcting malocclusions, preventing dental issues, and enhancing your child's facial appearance.

A CLOSER LOOK AT ORTHODONTIC APPLIANCES

Orthodontic appliances are pivotal in enhancing both facial aesthetics and respiratory well-being. They address misaligned bites, correct malocclusion, facilitate jaw expansion, and maintain post-treatment alignment—all contributing to improved breathing function and facial harmony. Early intervention during childhood offers significant advantages. Firstly, it promotes better dental health by proactively addressing misalignment and irregular bites and reducing the likelihood of cavities, gum disease, and other dental issues. This proactive approach lays the groundwork for long-term oral health. Secondly, it boosts self-esteem by addressing dental concerns early, minimizing potential self-consciousness, and cultivating confidence in one's smile and overall appearance.

Thirdly, early orthodontic treatment not only resolves current dental concerns but also prevents future complications. Guiding dental and jaw growth in youth helps avert severe issues like crowded teeth or overcrowding later on. This proactive approach diminishes the necessity for extensive orthodontic procedures in the future, hence saving time, expenses, and potential discomfort for the child.

Children can benefit from early intervention through different types of orthodontic treatments.

Headgear

Headgear is an orthodontic device that gently pulls on the upper teeth and jaw to treat severe bite issues. It facilitates the development of the upper jaw, which opens up the airway and can enhance facial appearance.

Braces and Aligners

These aim to correct misalignment issues in teeth and jaws. Traditional braces, consisting of brackets and wires, gradually align teeth while clear aligner therapy achieves similar results using removable trays. Clear aligners, made of transparent plastic, offer a discreet option for those who prefer less noticeable treatment. The smooth plastic feels more comfortable than traditional metal braces and allows for easier cleaning, as the trays can be removed for brushing and flossing. This convenience has led to increased adoption among both adults and children seeking improved hygiene during orthodontic treatment.

When it comes to airway health, braces and aligners can indirectly contribute to improving breathing patterns. If sleep apnea is linked to an overbite or misaligned teeth, orthodontists may recommend braces or aligners to address these underlying issues.

Palatal Expanders

Another orthodontic device used to enlarge the upper jaw is the palatal expander. In order to treat crowding or misalignment between the upper and lower jaws, palatal expanders are orthodontic devices that broaden the arch. A broader arch allows for more space for teeth to align properly, reducing crowding and overlapping in consequence. This can lead to better chewing efficiency and a more stable bite. Palatal expanders progressively widen the upper jaw by gently pressing on the upper teeth and the roof of the mouth. Because the roof of the mouth is the floor of the nose, this jaw enlargement improves and increases the amount of airflow being inhaled. Also, it improves the airflow across the nose. Improved nasal breathing can lessen mouth breathing-related problems like sleep apnea and snoring.

Retainers

Retainers play a vital role in preserving the results achieved with braces or aligners in orthodontic treatment by preventing teeth from shifting back to their original positions. Fixed retainers are customized wires bonded to the inside surfaces of teeth to maintain their corrected alignment while removable retainers, typically made of wire and plastic, can be easily taken out for cleaning and eating. Both types of retainers are essential for upholding the effectiveness of orthodontic treatment and ensuring lasting airway health by preventing teeth from relapsing.

Common Appliances for Specific Issues

Orthodontic appliances are crucial tools used by both orthodontists and general dentists to address specific dental issues. By applying targeted pressure to teeth and jaws, these appliances aim to gradually move them into proper alignment, thereby ensuring optimal functionality and appearance of the smile. There are various types of orthodontic appliances each serving unique purposes and offering different levels of flexibility and permanence in treatment. These include active appliances that actively move teeth and jaws into desired positions, passive appliances that maintain the achieved alignment, and both removable and fixed appliances offering different levels of convenience and permanence in treatment.

Active orthodontic appliances, such as the Mara and Forsus, are tailored to promote jaw growth and enhance facial structure by addressing overbites and improving jaw alignment in conjunction with traditional braces. Devices like the face mask specifically target underbites in growing children by advancing the upper jaw, potentially reducing the need for future jaw surgery. On the other hand, passive orthodontic appliances like the transpalatal arch (TPA) and lingual arch wire are critical for maintaining the position of teeth after orthodontic interventions such as palatal expansion or to compensate for early tooth loss, thus ensuring the longevity of the treatment results.

Removable orthodontic appliances, including elastics and the Sagittal Expander, offer the flexibility of correcting misalignments by applying controlled pressure to move teeth gradually. Elastics connect teeth in specific configurations, while expanders adjust the width of the upper jaw to relieve crowding. Meanwhile, fixed appliances such as temporary anchorage devices (TADs) and bite turbos provide a stable solution for complex dental issues by securing teeth in place to facilitate correct jaw development and protect other dental structures during treatment. Overall, orthodontic appliances offer diverse solutions for dental issues, therefore ensuring optimal outcomes and long-term oral health.

CASE STUDIES

Many children have used these appliances, hence significantly improving their quality of life. Take the following examples.

Andrew

Andrew faced a unique set of dental challenges including a crossbite and a family history of underbites coupled with premature gum recession. Determined to improve his situation, he embarked on an 8-month journey with an innovative treatment plan. This included the use of an expander and a face mask specifically designed to promote the forward growth of his upper jaw, thus correcting the crossbite and enhancing his facial profile. As the months progressed, not only did Andrew's crossbite resolve but his gum health also saw remarkable improvements. By the end of his treatment, Andrew had gained a more attractive smile and improvements to his oral health.

Kyle

Kyle's orthodontic adventure began with a challenging deep bite where his upper front teeth overlapped his lower ones more than usual—a trait he inherited from his family. To tackle this, he was fitted with braces and a custom bite plate designed to carefully lessen this overlap. Over 10 transformative months, these tools effectively corrected the deep bite and improved its functionality. Kyle witnessed remarkable improvements in both his dental alignment and the overall appeal of his facial profile.

Jack

Jack's journey to a better smile began with overcoming the challenges of an overbite—a condition worsened by his childhood thumb sucking. His treatment featured braces and strategic use of elastics aimed at not only enhancing his facial profile but also correcting the overbite and realigning his anterior teeth. Over the course of 10 transformative months, Jack's dedication paid off. His dental alignment and aesthetics improved dramatically leading to a more balanced and visually appealing smile that boosted his confidence and changed his outlook on life.

Catherine

Catherine's orthodontic journey not only reshaped her smile but also brought significant improvements to her overall oral health. Starting with a palatal expander, her treatment addressed her narrow upper palate and posterior crossbite— crucial steps for preventing future dental issues. As she transitioned to clear aligners, Catherine experienced a gradual enhancement in how her teeth functioned together including bite improvement and more comfortable eating. Over the course of 12 months, these changes not only perfected her teeth's alignment but also reduced the risk of tooth decay, contributing to her long-term health and well-being later on.

TIMING IS EVERYTHING

Orthodontic treatment plays a pivotal role in enhancing dental health and aesthetics, but the timing of when to start this treatment can significantly influence its effectiveness and outcome. Early intervention, often recommended during childhood or adolescence, can harness the natural growth processes to correct developmental anomalies. This preemptive approach not only addresses structural issues like misaligned jaws or crowded teeth more effectively but also potentially shortens the treatment duration and reduces the need for more invasive procedures later on. For adults, while treatment may take slightly longer due to matured bone structures, advancements in orthodontic technology continue to make it possible to achieve substantial improvements at any age.

One of the most transformative benefits of orthodontic treatment is the remarkable boost in confidence it offers, particularly to young patients navigating the challenges of growing up. A well-aligned smile can significantly enhance a child's self-esteem by empowering them to smile more freely and engage more confidently in social interactions. The inclusion of customizable appliances in their treatment plan— braces with changeable elastic colors or parts that glow in the dark or shine with glitter—adds an extra layer of excitement. These fun features not only personalize the experience but also make children look forward to their orthodontic appointments. By allowing kids to express their personality through their braces, orthodontic treatment becomes a more enjoyable and empowering journey deeply motivating them to participate actively in the process and embrace their improving smiles.

Another significant benefit of orthodontic treatment is its positive impact on speech development. Misaligned teeth can create difficulties with pronunciation leading to challenges in clear and effective communication. Correcting these dental irregularities through orthodontic interventions can open the door to clearer speech, ultimately enabling individuals to articulate words more precisely. This improvement can be particularly crucial during the formative years when children are mastering language skills. Enhanced speech not only boosts confidence but also facilitates better academic and social interactions. As children find it easier to express themselves, they become more engaged in conversations and active in classroom discussions, which paves the way for successful communication in their personal and future professional lives.

Orthodontic treatment does more than straighten teeth; it sets the stage for your child's healthy growth and development. By aligning the jaws and ensuring teeth are straight, it not only enables your child to chew food more effectively, which is crucial for good digestion and nutrient absorption, but it also helps teeth move smoothly into their ideal positions. This effective chewing can actually speed up the orthodontic process, especially during a growth spurt. In addition, a well-aligned set of teeth functions better and is easier to clean, therefore reducing the risk of trapped food particles and minimizing plaque buildup that can lead to tooth decay and gum disease.

Taking a proactive approach by guiding adult teeth into their proper positions while children wear braces is a strategic move in orthodontic care. This early intervention prepares the mouth for incoming adult teeth, therefore ensuring they align correctly and minimizing future dental issues. Braces correct existing problems and prevent future ones by adjusting the teeth and creating space, subsequently preventing overcrowding and misalignment as adult teeth emerge. Ultimately, careful management during a child's developmental years helps avoid more invasive and costly dental corrections in the future.

Furthermore, proper alignment intercepts and prevents skeletal jaw problems by ensuring that the bite functions as intended. This not only helps in distributing bite forces evenly and preventing excessive wear and tear on individual teeth but also reduces the strain on jaw muscles and joints. These orthodontic corrections can therefore significantly decrease the likelihood of developing chronic conditions such as TMJ disorders.

Additionally, if your child experiences recurring headaches or neck pain, it could be indicative of unnoticed teeth grinding. This condition often arises from a restricted airway exacerbated by factors like enlarged tonsils, or a misaligned jaw. Left unattended, grinding can lead to significant discomfort and potential complications. Orthodontic interventions offer a solution by realigning the jaw, alleviating symptoms, and preventing long-term issues. Addressing the root cause, whether it is jaw misalignment or airway obstruction, is pivotal for your child's overall well-being.

Another seemingless harmless habit that gets overlooked is thumb-sucking. It really does affect your child's smile if not tackled early. Ever noticed how thumb sucking seems to bring instant comfort to little ones? It is a natural reflex in early childhood that provides a sense of comfort and security. But did you know that letting this habit linger past the age of six can lead to serious dental issues? Things like misaligned teeth and changes in the shape of the palate can crop up. That is where braces swoop in as heroes. Not only do they straighten teeth but they also help kick those pesky habits like thumb sucking to the curb. Orthodontists might even suggest specialized appliances designed to stop thumb sucking and encourage healthier oral practices.

Your child can flash a confident smile knowing their teeth will stay beautiful to come. However, to keep those gains it is important to maintain tooth stability after orthodontic treatment. This is crucial for keeping your child's smile looking great and ensuring long-term oral health. Once the braces come off or aligners are no longer needed, teeth naturally want to shift back to their original positions—a phenomenon known as relapse. Here is the secret: retainers! These handy devices hold the teeth in their new, corrected positions, preventing unwanted movement as a result. Ensuring stability not only keeps the smile looking great but also plays a crucial role in maintaining proper dental alignment and functionality for years to come. By consistently using retainers and scheduling regular check-ups with a qualified dentist or orthodontist, you can protect the investment made in achieving a healthy, beautiful smile.

Taking action now by consulting with a dental professional is not just a choice for today; it is an investment in your child's future well-being and confidence. A beaming, confident grin awaits—do not let it slip away!

QUICK RECAP

- Ancient civilizations utilized rudimentary forms of braces to align teeth, even among the deceased, reflecting cultural beliefs about the importance of dental aesthetics in the afterlife.
- Orthodontic interventions extend beyond aesthetics to enhancing breathing patterns, such as through arch expansion, and promoting nasal breathing over mouth breathing for improved respiratory health.

- Orthodontic treatment not only corrects smiles but also fosters optimal airway development, thus reducing obstructions and risks of sleep disorders like sleep apnea.
- Orthodontic treatment can alleviate mouth breathing, counter OSA, and enhance sleep quality, thereby promoting better health.
- Orthodontics enhances facial structure by aligning teeth and jaws and correcting issues like underbites, overbites, and open bites for improved aesthetics and oral function.
- Various orthodontic appliances, such as braces, clear aligners, headgear, and expanders target specific issues like malocclusions, therefore contributing to improved airway health and facial harmony.
- Early orthodontic treatment offers benefits like boosting confidence, improving speech development, preventing future problems, and guiding proper jaw growth, ultimately supporting long-term oral health.

In the next chapter, you will learn about the essential role you play in influencing your children's habits. It will empower you with strategies to model and instill healthy habits in your family.

CHAPTER 9
A GOOD EXAMPLE

 *Your children will become what you are; so be
what you want them to be.*

DAVID BLY

LEADING YOUR BROOD

As a parent, you are the role model for your child's oral
health, and the way you care for your teeth and mouth
can have a profound impact on their habits and choices. Think
of your dental routine as a daily performance, and your child
as your biggest fan closely observing and emulating your
every move. When you brush and floss regularly, you are
painting a picture of good habits that they are likely to follow.

By turning dental care into a family adventure and making it
fun, you can create a sense of excitement around oral hygiene.
When you cheer them on for brushing well or praise them for

flossing, you are not just encouraging a behavior; you are showing them that oral health is important. On the flip side, if you neglect your own dental care, your child might think it is not a big deal either.

Your attitude toward the dentist can set the stage for your child's feelings as well. If you are nervous or anxious about dental visits, they might inherit that fear, making check-ups a dreaded event as a result.

By making dental hygiene a family priority, you are laying the groundwork for a lifetime of healthy habits and beautiful smiles. It is an investment in their future well-being, and with your encouragement, they will have the confidence to keep up the great work.

The Role of Parents in Setting Examples for Healthy Living

Parents, you play a big role in showing your children how to live healthy lives. What you eat, how you stay active, and how you handle stress all influence your children. They watch and learn from you, so when you make healthy choices you are teaching them to do the same.

But it is not just about what you do; it is also about what you say and how you talk about healthy living. Talking openly about eating well, exercising, and why it is important helps your children understand why these things matter. When you make healthy activities like cooking together or playing outside part of your family routine, you are showing them that these habits are important for staying healthy in the long run.

On the other hand, if you spend too much time on screens or eat lots of unhealthy food, your children might pick up those habits too. So, it is important to be mindful of your own actions because they can shape your child's future.

Encouraging Healthy Choices and Good Habits

While parents play a big role in teaching their children to make good choices, it takes more than just showing them how. It is important to create an environment that supports them, lets them make their own decisions, and teaches them to be responsible. Here is how you can do that:

- **Lead by example:** Be the superhero of your child's health! By taking care of yourself, you show your children how to be healthy too. Let them see you brushing your teeth, eating nutritious foods, and staying active to keep your body strong and vibrant. Your actions speak louder than words, and when they see you living a healthy lifestyle, they will want to do the same.
- **Explain the benefits:** Tell your children why it is so important to take care of their teeth and body. You can frame it as a mini-science lesson or a story; explain that if they do not brush properly, they might get cavities or sore gums that can hurt. This way, they understand that keeping their mouth clean and healthy is not just a chore—it is essential for their well-being.
- **Make it fun:** Transform brushing and flossing into a delightful adventure! Use colorful toothbrushes,

yummy-flavored toothpaste and fun games to make cleaning their teeth exciting. You can even make up a catchy song or create a brushing challenge to see who can clean their teeth the best.

- **Set a routine:** Create a daily schedule for brushing teeth and other healthy activities and stick to it. Make sure your children know what they need to do each day to keep their teeth and body healthy. This routine helps establish good habits and makes health a consistent priority in their lives.

- **Reward good habits:** Celebrate their successes! When your children do a great job taking care of their teeth, tell them how proud you are and maybe give them a little treat or praise. Positive reinforcement helps them remember to keep up the good work and makes oral care a natural, enjoyable habit.

Take for example Sarah and her daughter Emily—both my patients. From the moment Emily was a toddler, Sarah treated oral hygiene like a treasured family ritual. She showed Emily how to brush her teeth properly, made regular trips to the dentist a priority, and always emphasized the importance of caring for their teeth.

As Emily grew up, these habits became a natural part of her daily routine even when she left for college. She realized her mom had armed her with the tools to keep her smile bright and healthy. Reflecting on her childhood, Emily felt immense gratitude for her mom's guidance and knew she wanted to pass on these valuable lessons to her own children one day.

Meanwhile, Michael—another one of my patients—grew up in a household where fast food and sugary snacks were the norm. Picture a kitchen table laden with burgers, fries, and candy—a tempting yet harmful feast. This environment shaped Michael's taste buds and habits steering him toward unhealthy choices. Despite efforts to educate him about the benefits of nutritious eating, Michael found it tough to break free from the patterns he learned at home.

As an adult, Michael battles with weight issues and other health challenges—shadows from his upbringing that linger on. These contrasting stories highlight how parents' influence on their children's habits can impact them for a lifetime. It is a poignant reminder that the lessons we learn early on, like seeds planted in fertile soil, can grow into lasting patterns— whether beneficial or detrimental.

BREATHWORK FOR PARENTS: ENHANCING YOUR OWN HEALTH

Michael had often felt overwhelmed and stressed due to his health issues. As he grapples with weight problems and other challenges stemming from his upbringing, I have encouraged him to try something simple yet transformative: breathing exercises. As adults, we often forget that something as simple as breathing can have a profound impact on our well-being. Even for those with the busiest schedules, these exercises offer unique benefits whether it is energizing you for the day ahead, calming your mind before bed, or simply helping you stay present in the moment. In addition to diaphragmatic, bee, and box breathing, here are some techniques you can try out.

Bellows Breath

When feeling overwhelmed by endless to-dos and sleep deprivation, the bellows breath technique can offer a revitalizing boost. This energizing practice ignites focus and clarity amidst chaos like a reset for your mind. It enhances digestion, metabolism, and mental acuity, empowering you to tackle challenges with renewed vigor as a consequence.

To perform the bellows breath, sit comfortably with your elbows bent and hands at shoulder height while forming fists with your palms facing inward. Spread your fingers wide and lift your arms overhead as you inhale deeply through your nose. Then, exhale forcefully and swiftly through your nose as you bring your arms back down to shoulder height with closed fists. Repeat this process 10 times, then relax and breathe normally. It is wise to avoid this exercise on a full stomach.

Resonance breathing

Resonance breathing, also known as coherent breathing, is a deeply relaxing technique that calms by synchronizing your breathing with your heart rate. It is a wonderful tool for busy individuals seeking a peaceful moment in their day to manage stress. Sit or lie down comfortably—spine straight. Close your eyes and breathe in slowly through your nose for a count of five. Then, exhale gently through your nose for a count of five. Continue this pattern aiming for five breaths per minute as you focus on the soothing rhythm of your breath.

Adding breathing exercises to your daily routine can truly be a game-changer for you and your loved ones. These simple practices offer a multitude of benefits from lowering blood pressure to sharpening focus. They can also spark creativity by clearing your mind of distractions and inviting fresh ideas to flourish without the interference of mental clutter. Plus, when your little ones witness you taking charge of your well-being and staying cool under pressure, you are not just setting an example; you are showing them how to thrive. And as you prioritize your well-being, you naturally deepen your connections with loved ones and foster a sense of unity and harmony within your family circle. Feel free to share these exercises with others, you are not just helping yourself—you are paving the way for a happier, more mindful future for everyone you care about.

POSTURE FOR PARENTS

But here is the kicker: good posture can supercharge the effects of breathing exercises. When you stand or sit up straight, it helps your lungs take in more air making each breath count. Conversely, poor posture can lead to a host of issues from muscle imbalances to nagging back pain that make it harder to breathe deeply. Worse yet, this can affect how you play and interact with your kids. By honing your posture, you are not just optimizing your breathing—you are also showing your kids the importance of taking care of themselves. Additionally, the perks of good posture extend far beyond physical health. It boosts confidence, elevates mood, and minimizes the risk of enduring discomfort, therefore ensuring you can keep pace with your little ones effortlessly.

Common Posture Issues Faced by Adults

Developing bad posture can happen without much conscious thought. Think of your body as a tall, proud building. Without even realizing it, you gradually might start to slouch or lean forward, especially if you spend a lot of time looking at your phone or sitting in a chair. Carrying a heavy backpack or repeating the same motions at work can also make your posture worse.

Other things like being overweight, pregnant, or wearing shoes that do not fit right can affect your posture too. Even having one leg slightly shorter than the other or a condition called scoliosis—lateral curving and rotation of the spine— can make you stand or walk a bit crooked.

All these things can slowly change how you hold yourself and pull you out of your optimal alignment. Recognizing these factors is the first step toward fixing your posture and standing tall again.

Forward head

Forward head posture is like carrying a heavy load perpetually balanced on your neck and shoulders. Imagine your head as a bowling ball that is always leaning forward thus putting strain on your muscles and ligaments at the back of your neck and spine. This posture often develops from spending long hours hunched over computers or smartphones causing the neck to extend unnaturally as if reaching towards the screen. Over time, this can lead to muscle strain, discomfort, and even chronic pain, as the body struggles to support the forward shift of its natural balance. As you age, muscle strength in your upper body may diminish contributing to forward head posture. Correcting this posture involves regular awareness of your head position, strengthening exercises for the neck and upper back, and making ergonomic adjustments to your workspace to support a more aligned posture.

Swayback

Swayback posture involves an exaggerated inward curve in the lower back making the hips and stomach push forward while the upper back leans back. It is like your body is mimicking a relaxed, reclining position even while standing. This misalignment often develops from poor sitting habits, weak core muscles, or imbalances in muscle strength and flexibility. Over time, swayback can lead to discomfort and pain in the lower back and legs as the body compensates for its shifted center of gravity. To correct swayback, strengthening the abdominal and gluteal muscles along with practicing exercises that promote better pelvic alignment are essential steps. Additionally, becoming more conscious of maintaining a neutral spine throughout the day can help in reducing this posture issue.

Kyphosis

Kyphosis involves an excessive outward curvature of the upper back creating a pronounced rounded appearance often referred to as a hunchback. It often arises from habits like slouching over screens, but age plays a role too. For instance, osteoporosis—thinning and weakening of bones—particularly affects older women and can exacerbate kyphosis. Additionally, the degeneration of spinal discs or vertebrae as people age can contribute to its development. In children, causes of kyphosis can include diseases like polio or Scheuermann's disease as well as the impact of undergoing treatments like chemotherapy or radiation for cancer. Addressing kyphosis often involves strengthening the back muscles, improving flexibility, and maintaining a more upright posture during daily activities.

Flatback

Flatback syndrome occurs when the natural curve of the lower spine flattens, therefore pushing sufferers into a perpetual forward lean. This unusual stance often leads to awkward compensations like bending the knees or craning the neck. Initially linked to spinal surgery outcomes, flatback can also arise from muscle imbalances or prolonged poor posture. Those affected may experience chronic back pain and fatigue, as they struggle daily to find balance. Effective treatments typically involve targeted physical therapy and exercises designed to strengthen and restore the spine's natural arc.

Other forms of posture involve:

- **Poking chin:** This posture emerges when the chin juts forward, subsequently misaligning the head with the neck and spine. Often due to prolonged screen use at improper heights, it strains the neck muscles and can lead to tension headaches.

- **Uneven shoulders or hips:** This posture imbalance where one shoulder or hip is higher than the other, can stem from habitual activities like always carrying a bag on one side or favoring one leg while standing. Over time, this asymmetry can cause discomfort and uneven wear on joints and muscles.
- **Military-style posture:** Characterized by a very straight back and squared shoulders, this posture might look healthy but can be problematic. Holding the body too rigid can strain the back and limit natural movements leading to muscle fatigue and tension.

Effects of bad posture

Did you know that the average person spends about 12 h a day sitting? This modern lifestyle habit can severely affect your posture leading to a range of health issues. Bad posture does more than just lead to aches and pains; it profoundly impacts your overall health. When you slouch or hunch, not only do your neck, shoulders, and back suffer but also your internal organs get compressed. This compression can disrupt your breathing and digestion making your body less efficient at its basic functions. Moreover, poor posture can influence your mood and energy levels often leading to feelings of lethargy and irritability. Over time, persistent bad posture can result in serious, long-term health issues like chronic pain, spinal problems, and reduced mobility. This is why it is crucial to stay mindful of your posture; correcting it can be a key step towards maintaining both physical and mental well-being. The good news is that improving your posture is achievable through targeted exercises like the ones below alongside the abovementioned downward facing dog.

Child's pose

Child's pose is an effective yoga position for enhancing posture and releasing tension in the back and neck. To perform it, start by sitting on your shins with knees together, toes touching, and heels spread apart. From this position, walk your hands forward as you hinge at the hips lowering your torso between your thighs. Allow your forehead to rest gently on the ground or turn your head to one side, and extend your arms forward or rest them by your sides. Placing a pillow under your thighs can offer additional support if needed. While in this pose, focus on deep, steady breathing filling your lower back and ribs with air. Holding this pose for five minutes can greatly aid in stretching your spine, glutes, and hamstrings while helping to soothe your mind and alleviate stress.

Forward fold

The forward fold is a classic yoga pose that offers multiple benefits, particularly for those looking to improve flexibility and relieve stress. To perform a forward fold, start by standing with feet hip-width apart. As you exhale, hinge at the hips and bend forward keeping the spine long. Allow your hands to fall towards the ground thus touching your feet, shins, or the mat depending on your flexibility. Your head should hang heavily adding a gentle stretch to your neck. This pose helps stretch the hamstrings and calves, and can also help relieve tension in the spine. The forward fold is not only great for improving flexibility but also encourages blood flow to the brain, accordingly calming the mind and reducing stress. It is a simple yet profoundly effective posture for enhancing overall well-being.

Cat-cow

The cat-cow stretch is a fluid movement that enhances spinal flexibility and promotes relaxation while improving blood circulation. To perform this exercise, begin on your hands and knees in a tabletop position ensuring your knees are set directly below your hips and your wrists, elbows, and shoulders are in line and perpendicular to the floor. For the "cow" part, inhale as you drop your belly towards the mat, lift your chin and chest, and gaze up toward the ceiling. Then, transition into "cat" by exhaling and drawing your belly to your spine and rounding your back toward the ceiling like a cat stretching. Regularly practicing cat-cow can help stretch and mobilize the spine, relieve tension in the torso, and calm the mind. Repeat this sequence smoothly for at least one minute to maximize its benefits.

Standing cat-cow

The standing cat-cow is a versatile adaptation of the traditional cat-cow stretch designed to be performed while standing. This variation is particularly beneficial for those who find floor exercises challenging or for a quick stretch during a work break. To begin, stand with your feet hip-width apart and place your hands on your knees. As you inhale, arch your back, push your abdomen forward, and lift your head and tailbone towards the ceiling to embody the cow position. As you exhale, round your spine outward, tuck your tailbone, and drop your head towards your chest mimicking the cat position. This exercise helps to mobilize the spine and can relieve tension in the back and neck. It also promotes flexibility and improves circulation making it a fantastic choice for maintaining spinal health and alleviating stiffness throughout the day.

Chest opener

If you find yourself sitting for long periods throughout the day, then the chest opener exercise is a beneficial way to relieve upper body tension. Start by standing with your feet about hip-width apart. Place your hands behind your back and interlace them by squeezing the palms together; if your hands cannot reach each other, you can use a towel to bridge the gap. Ensure you maintain proper alignment with your neck, spine, and head looking straight ahead. As you inhale, lift your chest and gently pull your hands towards the floor, hence deepening the stretch across your chest. Hold this position for about five deep breaths focusing on expanding your chest with each inhale. After holding, relax and take a few breaths before repeating. Performing this stretch at least 10 times can significantly open and stretch the chest muscles, improve posture, and promote deeper breathing—ideal for counteracting the stresses of prolonged desk work or driving.

High plank

The high plank is a foundational yoga pose that strengthens your shoulders, glutes, and hamstrings but also reduces pain and stiffness across the body. Start in a standing position and bend forward to place your hands flat on the ground shoulder-width apart. Step your feet back until your body forms a straight line from your heels to your head similar to the top of a push-up. Ensure your wrists are directly under your shoulders and engage your abdominal muscles to keep your torso steady. Avoid letting your hips sag or pike up, as maintaining a level position is crucial for activating the correct muscle groups. Hold this position for up to a minute while focusing on deep, even breaths to help maintain balance and strength. High plank not only builds physical strength but also enhances mental endurance, making it a versatile exercise for overall fitness in the long run.

Thoracic spine rotation

Thoracic spine rotation is a fundamental exercise for enhancing flexibility and mobility in the mid-back region. It is beneficial for individuals of all ages and activity levels, particularly those who spend long hours sitting or engaging in activities that promote a rounded posture. Office workers, athletes, fitness enthusiasts, and individuals experiencing back stiffness or discomfort can benefit from incorporating thoracic spine rotation into their routine. To perform this movement, begin in a seated position with legs crossed or extended comfortably. Place your hands behind your head keeping elbows wide and engage your core for stability. Slowly rotate your torso to one side leading with your chest while keeping hips squared. Hold the stretch briefly focusing on deep breathing to encourage relaxation. Return to the starting position and repeat on the opposite side for a balanced stretch. Repeat this movement 5–10 times remembering to alternate sides each time to ensure balanced flexibility and strength development across your thoracic spine.

Glute bridge

The glute bridge exercise offers numerous benefits, particularly for those seeking to improve lower body strength and address the effects of prolonged sitting. It effectively activates and strengthens muscles that may become weakened or inactive due to sedentary lifestyles. Additionally, it can help alleviate lower back discomfort and support individuals recovering from injuries. To perform a glute bridge, begin by lying on your back with knees bent and feet flat on the floor hip-width apart. Engage your core to stabilize your spine, then press through your heels to lift your hips off the ground while creating a straight line from shoulders to knees. Squeeze your glutes at the top, then lower your hips back down with control focusing on maintaining proper form and avoiding excessive arching of the lower back. Hold the lifted position for up to 1 min, as you ensure your shoulders remain grounded. This exercise enhances hip and pelvic function contributing to improved posture and overall alignment.

Isometric pulls

This is a versatile exercise suitable for a wide range of individuals, particularly those seeking to strengthen their upper body and improve posture. Isometric pulls involve holding a static position, which helps develop muscular endurance and promote joint stability. To perform this exercise, start by sitting comfortably in a chair with a soft backrest for support. Make a fist with each hand and extend your arms straight out in front of you ensuring they are parallel to the floor. Next, squeeze your shoulder blades together and draw your elbows back towards your shoulders exhaling as you do so. Hold this position for about 10 s while maintaining deep breathing. Inhale slowly as you release back to the starting position. Repeat this movement for approximately 1 min while focusing on maintaining proper form and engaging your upper back muscles throughout.

Just as you engage your muscles during exercise to promote strength and stability, ensuring your workspace is ergonomically optimized can help reduce discomfort in your neck, back, and wrists during long hours of work.

Start by adjusting your chair to ensure proper lumbar support and a comfortable height that allows your feet to rest flat on the floor or on a footrest. Position your desk at elbow height to maintain a neutral wrist position while typing. Keep enough space under your desk for your legs and try to keep it tidy to avoid clutter. Adjust the height of your desk if possible, and add something sturdy underneath to make it higher if needed. Cover sharp edges to protect your wrists.

Opt for an ergonomic keyboard and mouse to minimize strain on your wrists and forearms. Your hands should be at the same height as your elbows or a little lower.

Adjust your monitor so that the top of the screen is at or slightly below eye level to reduce neck strain. If using a laptop, consider using a separate keyboard and mouse to achieve a more ergonomic setup. Keep frequently used items within easy reach to minimize excessive reaching and twisting. If you frequently use a telephone, consider using the speaker mode or headset to avoid cradling the phone between your ear and shoulder, which can lead to neck discomfort.

As you fine-tune your workspace for comfort and efficiency, consider the ripple effect it can have beyond your desk. Your dedication to maintaining good posture is not just about personal health—it is a powerful lesson in self-care that echoes throughout your household. Envision a home where everyone embodies strength and vitality, where sitting with confidence is a shared principle rather than just a routine. Together, you are not just setting up ergonomic chairs and adjusting monitor heights; you are creating a culture of wellness. It is about instilling values that extend far beyond the workspace and shaping a future where strength, confidence, and healthy habits are second nature. So, as you engage in these exercises and settle into your ergonomic setup, remember that you are not just investing in your own comfort; you are nurturing a legacy where health and vitality flourish within your family.

QUICK RECAP

- Parental influence significantly impacts a child's oral health habits and overall lifestyle choices.
- Children observe, mimic, and internalize their parents' actions, including oral hygiene practices.
- Positive reinforcement and encouragement from parents are vital for promoting good oral health habits in children.
- Parents' attitudes towards dental care shape their children's perceptions and beliefs about oral hygiene.
- By actively involving children in oral care routines and making dental hygiene a family priority, parents establish a foundation for lifelong healthy habits.
- Parents serve as crucial role models for overall healthy living influencing not just oral health but broader lifestyle choices for their children.
- Effective parenting strategies involve creating a supportive environment that promotes autonomy, instilling a sense of responsibility, and providing resources and guidance for healthy habits.

In conclusion, prioritizing oral hygiene, healthy lifestyle choices, effective breathing techniques, and good posture not only benefits you but also sets impactful examples for your children, consequently promoting lifelong habits that contribute to their overall health and confidence.

AIRWAY DEVELOPMENT 101:

A BEGINNER'S GUIDE TO IMPROVING BREATHING, SLEEP QUALITY, AND ORAL HEALTH FOR YOU AND YOUR CHILDREN WITHOUT COMPLICATED TECHNIQUES

Now you have everything you need to achieve optimal airway health, it's time to pass on your newfound knowledge and show other readers where they can find the same help.

Simply by leaving your honest opinion of this book on Amazon, you'll show other parents and healthcare professionals where they can find the information they're looking for, and pass their passion for improved airway development forward.

Thank you for your help. Improved airway development is kept alive when we pass on our knowledge – and you're helping me to do just that.

Scan the QR code below:

Your review can help others breathe better, sleep soundly, and live healthier lives. Thank you for being a part of this journey.

Sincerely,

Dr. Markus Wilson

CONCLUSION

Throughout this book, we have delved deeply into the essentials of respiratory health, sleep quality, and oral well-being revealing how historical trends, personal habits, and lifestyle choices intertwine to influence our overall health. By weaving together a narrative that is both insightful and thorough, this book sheds light on how these elements not only shape our day-to-day wellness but also impact the long-term health of future generations.

At its heart, *Airway Development 101* is designed to empower you with practical knowledge and tools that enhance your well-being and that of your children. You have gained insights into identifying and addressing the signs of respiratory disorders, grasped the critical importance of early interventions for supporting healthy speech and facial development, and explored targeted breathing exercises suitable for various ages. Moreover, you have discovered the profound effects that everyday lifestyle choices can have on respiratory health equipping you with the information needed to make informed decisions that promote healthier living.

We have also unpacked the crucial link between nutrition, oral health, and optimal airway function by demonstrating how these factors are interconnected with the quality of sleep and overall respiratory health. With this understanding, you are now better equipped to pinpoint sleep-related breathing issues and to create an environment that promotes restful sleep for both you and your family.

Moreover, we have explored the impactful role of orthodontics in airway development through highlighting how timely orthodontic interventions can significantly benefit your children's respiratory health. Most importantly, you have learned about the critical role parents play in setting examples and fostering healthy habits at home. These habits extend beyond mere physical health—they enhance vitality, boost cognitive function, and elevate the overall quality of life. Through this knowledge, you are empowered to lay a strong foundation for lifelong wellness for your entire family.

Amidst the uncertainty and despair of my personal journey, there came a turning point—a revelation that would change the course of my health journey. After a long struggle and determined self-advocacy, my parents and I finally connected with a medical professional who truly understood the severity of my condition and provided a solution. The treatment— removing my enlarged tonsils and orthodontic care—opened up a new chapter in my life marked by significant emotional and physical relief.

This change brought an incredible transformation. The overwhelming exhaustion I used to feel was lifted and replaced by a vibrant sense of vitality. Nights were no longer filled with dread, and mornings felt refreshing and energetic rather than more tired than when I had gone to bed. The gradually disappearing bags under my eyes were replaced by the glow of restful sleep. It was a transformation that extended beyond the physical realm eventually permeating every aspect of my life.

This personal journey underscores the importance of awareness and early intervention in health matters—a theme that echoes throughout this book. By sharing my story, I aim to encourage you to recognize the signs and symptoms of airway issues, take charge of your health, and seek the support you need.

As you turn the final page of this chapter, remember that the power to improve your own health or that of your children rests in your hands. Seize this opportunity to take charge by starting with small, manageable steps toward healthier habits. Whether it is adding breathing exercises to your daily routine, enhancing your sleep hygiene, or prioritizing nutritious meals, every action you take contributes to improving your airway.

Keep in mind that the earlier you start, the greater the impact will be. Your commitment to health will not only benefit you but also inspire those around you to follow suit. So, why wait? Take that first step today and embark on your path to a healthier, happier life.

I also invite you to share your journey and insights by leaving a review. Your feedback does more than inform—it ignites the transformative potential of this story and supports the author's mission to empower individuals and families across the globe. By leaving your review, you become part of the legacy of this narrative by contributing to its lasting impact on the lives it touches and the generations to come. Embrace this journey toward health and vitality, and let every breath you take be a testament to the power of informed, proactive living.

REFERENCES

A parent's guide to proper breathing. (2023, March 15). CAFF. *https://www. childrensairwayfirst.org/post/a-parent-s-guide-to-proper-breathing*

Allergic rhinitis in children. (n.d.). Hopkins Medicine. *https://www. hopkinsmedicine.org/health/conditions-and-diseases/allergic-rhinitis-in-children*

Amanda L., C. (2011, November 25). *A possible reason for overcrowded teeth.* HuffPost. *https://www.huffpost.com/entry/overcrowded-teeth-eating-habits-evolution_n_1110992*

Anderson, P. (2021, April 8). *What age should children start myofunctional therapy?* MyoMatters. *https://www.myomatters.com/post/what-age-should-children-start-myofunctional-therapy*

Ankrom, S. (2023, January 27). *Nine breathing exercises to relieve anxiety.* Verywell Mind. *https://www.verywellmind.com/abdominal-breathing-2584115*

Ankush, K. (2021, March 25). *Twelve enormous benefits of early orthodontic treatment for your kids.* Fresh Orthodontics. *https://www.freshorthodontics. com/12-enormous-benefits-of-early-orthodontic-treatment-for-your-kids*

Ardeshna, T. (2022, April 21). *The role of nutrition in facial formation and breathing.* TruCare Dentistry Roswell.*https://www.trucaredentistry.com/ blog/the-role-of-nutrition-in-facial-formation-and-breathing*

Baby-led weaning (BLW): A complete guide to first foods. (2024, April 10). Huckleberry. *https://huckleberrycare.com/blog/baby-led-weaning*

Beck, C. (2023, April 17). *Posture exercises for kids.* The OT Toolbox. *https:// www.theottoolbox.com/posture-exercises-for-kids*

Benefits of omega-3 fatty acid for oral health. (n.d.). Mint Kids Dentistry. *https://www.mintkidsdentistry.com/b/benefits-of-omega-3-fatty-acid-for-oral-health*

Benefits of zinc for bad breath & oral health. (2017, October 17). SmartMouth. *https://smartmouth.com/blog/zinc-oral-health/*

Breastfeeding is good for oral and oro-facial health. (2020, January 20). Grand Lake Dental. *https://www.grandlakedental.com/blog/2020/1/20/ breastfeeding-is-good-for-oral-and-oro-facial-health*

Breathing. (2014, August 20). The Lung Association. *https://www.lung.ca/ lung-health/lung-info/breathing*

Brody, B. (2022). *When is it time for my baby to use a cup instead of a bottle?* WebMD. *https://www.webmd.com/parenting/baby/features/bottle-to-cup*

Bulmash, T. (2017, August 29). *Six easy ways to improve your child's posture*. Body and Posture LCC. *https://www.bodyandposture.com/single-post/2017/ 08/29/6-easy-ways-to-improve-your-childs-posture*

Can braces open an airway? (2022, September 12). Dental Hygiene Resource. *https://www.dentalhygiene411.com/holistic-health/can-braces-open-an- airway*

Cherney, K. (2019, December 16). *Do air purifiers work? Research, best practices, and more*. Healthline. *https://www.healthline.com/health/ allergies/do-air-purifiers-work*

Cherry, K. (2007, June 16). *The 4 stages of sleep (NREM and REM Sleep Cycles)*. Verywell Health. *https://www.verywellhealth.com/the-four-stages- of-sleep-2795920*

Clare, W. (2021, November 20). *Canine teeth shrank in human ancestors at least 4.5 million years ago*. New Scientist. *https://www.newscientist.com/ article/2299286-canine-teeth-shrank-in-human-ancestors-at-least-4-5- million-years-ago/*

Clark, L. (2015, February 16). *Before agriculture, human jaws were a perfect fit for human teeth*. MyBib. *https://www.mybib.com/#/projects/GG1G1z/ citations*

Cleft lip and cleft palate: Causes, diagnosis & treatment. (2022, June 13). Cleveland Clinic. *https://my.clevelandclinic.org/health/diseases/10947- cleft-lip-cleft-palate*

Cronkleton, E. (2018). *Posture exercises: 12 exercises to improve your posture*. Healthline. *https://www.healthline.com/health/posture-exercises*

Cronkleton, E. (2019, April 9). *Ten breathing techniques*. Healthline. *https:// www.healthline.com/health/breathing-exercise*

Cucuzzella, Ambrose, S. (n.d.). How do your lungs work? Scientific American. https://www.scientificamerican.com/article/how-do-your-lungs-work/

Dando, J., & Fricker, J. (n.d.). *Mouth breathing*. ScienceDirect. *https://www. sciencedirect.com/topics/medicine-and-dentistry/mouth-breathing*

Darendeliler, A., & Kharbanda, O. P. (2016). *Long face syndrome*. ScienceDirect. *https://www.sciencedirect.com/topics/medicine-and- dentistry/long-face-syndrome*

Delayed tooth eruption: Should my child see a dentist? (2020, July 8). Woodhill Dental Specialties. *https://www.woodhilldentalspecialties.com/*

delayed-tooth-eruption-what-to-expect/

Dental and oral anatomy. (2019). UpToDate. https://www.uptodate.com/contents/dental-and-oral-anatomy

Deviated septum: Symptoms and causes. (2019). Mayo Clinic. *https://www.mayoclinic.org/diseases-conditions/deviated-septum/symptoms-causes/syc-20351710*

Doman, E. (2016, May 23). *How hypoallergenic bedding can help you sleep.* Allergy and Air. *https://learn.allergyandair.com/hypoallergenic-bedding-and-sleep/*

Dr Ross Orthodontics Team. (2022, October 27). *Three ways your child's breathing can improve with orthodontic treatments.* David Ross Orthodontics. *https://davidrossorthodontics.com/3-ways-your-childs-breathing-can-improve-with-orthodontic-treatments*

Duty, S. (2020, January 6). *Children's dentist explains: The effects of sugar on your child's teeth.* Smiles Dentistry 4 Kids. *https://smilesdentistry4kids.com/childrens-dentist-explains-the-effects-of-sugar-on-your-childs-teeth*

Enlarged tonsils. (n.d.). Nationwide Children's. *https://www.nationwidechildrens.org/conditions/enlarged-tonsils*

Enlarged tonsils and adenoids: Overview. (2019). Institute for Quality and Efficiency in Health Care (IQWiG). *https://www.ncbi.nlm.nih.gov/books/NBK536881/*

Everything you need to know about airway anatomy. (2023, May 11). Bloom. *https://bloomsleepandairway.com/2023/05/11/airway-anatomy-everything-you-need-to-know/*

Exercise to build healthy lungs. (2022). My Health. *https://www.myhealth.va.gov/mhv-portal-web/ss20181019-build-healthy-lungs*

Fifteen breathwork benefits: The science behind breathing practices. (n.d.). Other Ship. *https://www.othership.us/resources/breathwork-benefits*

Five advantages of nose breathing. (2021, October 27). Modern Family Dental Care. *https://modernfamilydentalcare.com/5-advantages-of-nose-breathing*

Gonzalez, D. (2016, June 26). *Ten posture myths everyone should know.* Family Health Chiropractic. *https://www.familyhealthchiropractic.com/10-posture-myths-everyone-know*

Gordon, S. (2022, November 9). *How to get your child to stop sucking their thumb.* Verywell Family. *https://www.verywellfamily.com/how-to-stop-thumb-sucking-in-kids-4158357*

Gupta, P. (2016, January 20). *Five techniques for tongue aerobics.* 1SpecialPlace. *https://www.1specialplace.com/2016/01/21/tongue-aerobics/*

How airway orthodontics can help your child? (2019, October 18). Adventure

Orthodontics. https://www.adventureortho.com/understanding-how-airway-orthodontics-can-help-your-child/

How calcium plays a crucial role in oral health. (2021). Delta Dental. *https://www1.deltadentalins.com/wellness/nutrition/articles/calcium*

How does shallow breathing impact your life. (n.d.). Awakened Mind. *https://awakenedmind.com/Insights/52/How-does-shallow-breathing-impact-your-life*

How many breaths do you take each day? (n.d.). Wonderopolis. *https://wonderopolis.org/wonder/how-many-breaths-do-you-take-each-day*

How poor nutrition affects your oral health. (2023, April 28). ProHEALTH Dental. *https://www.phdental.com/oral-health-news/2023/april/how-poor-nutrition-affects-your-oral-health/*

How to enhance symmetry and beauty naturally. (n.d.). Kion. *https://www.getkion.com/blogs/all/super-model*

How your child's nutrition can affect their oral health. (n.d.). Hometown Family Dental. *https://www.hometownfamilydentalnc.com/blog/how-your-childs-nutrition-can-affect-their-oral-health*

Human history in your face. (2019, April 23). Earthsky. *https://earthsky.org/human-world/how-why-human-face-evolved-to-look-as-it-does-today*

Humidifiers: Why you might need them. (2019). Mayo Clinic. *https://www.mayoclinic.org/diseases-conditions/common-cold/in-depth/humidifiers/art-20048021*

Improving your child's oral health with myofunctional therapy. (n.d.). Tompkins Dental. *https://www.tompkinsdental.com/blog/improving-your-childs-oral-health-with-myofunctional-therapy*

Jaw and facial development in children. (n.d.). Apex Dental. https://apexdentaliowa.com/jaw-and-facial-development-in-children/

Joseph M., D. (2022, March 21). *Vitamin C and your oral health.* Dr. Joe's Blog. https://www.drdalbon.com/for-our-patients/dr-joe_s-blog/2022/3/21/vitamin-c-and-your-oral-health

Kivi, R. (2018, March 26). *What Causes an airway obstruction, and how is it treated?* Healthline. https://www.healthline.com/health/airway-obstruction

Knapp, W. (2023, June 8). *Nine ways to create the best ergonomic workstation setup.* Weber Knapp. *https://blog.weberknapp.com/tips-for-an-ergonomic-workstation-setup*

Kovar, E. (2015, November 2). *How posture affects breathing.* ACE Fitness. https://www.acefitness.org/resources/everyone/blog/5716/how-posture-affects-breathing

Leszczyszyn, A., Hnitecka, S., & Dominiak, M. (2021). Could vitamin D3 deficiency influence malocclusion development? *Nutrients, 13(6),* 2122. https://doi.org/10.3390/nu13062122

Linda. (2022, April 29). *What vitamins & minerals benefit your oral health?* Complete Dental Works. https://completedentalworks.com.au/what-vitamins-minerals-benefit-your-oral-health/

Long-face syndrome: What is it and how is it treated. (2019, June 12). Instituto Maxilofacial. *https://www.institutomaxilofacial.com/en/2019/06/12/long-face-syndrome-what-is-it-and-how-is-it-treated*

Magnesium for your brain and mouth health. (2023, May 10). Dental Wellness. https://dentalwellness.com.au/magnesium-for-your-brain-and-mouth-health

Maypole, M. (2018, June 12). *Eight ways to help your child get rid of the pacifier.* Healthline. https://www.healthline.com/health/baby/how-to-get-rid-of-the-pacifier

McKeown, P. (n.d.). *Nose breathing vs mouth breathing: Benefits, sleep, science.* Oxygen Advantage. https://oxygenadvantage.com/science/nose-breathing-vs-mouth-breathing

Mechanics of breathing. (n.d.). TeachMePhysiology. https://teachmephysiology.com/respiratory-system/ventilation/mechanics-of-breathing

Michael D. B., & Moore, J. (2016). *Fluctuating asymmetry.* ScienceDirect. https://www.sciencedirect.com/topics/medicine-and-dentistry/fluctuating-asymmetry

Mindful breathing for kids, teens and the young at heart. (2021, March 18). Back on Track Teens. https://www.backontrackteens.com/blog/mindful-breathing-for-kids-teens-and-the-young-at-heart/

Myofunctional issues in children aged 2-5. (2016, September 8). KidsTown Dental. https://kidstowndentist.com/myofunctional-issues-children-aged-2-5/

Nasal polyps: Symptoms and causes. (2019). Mayo Clinic. https://www.mayoclinic.org/diseases-conditions/nasal-polyps/symptoms-causes/syc-20351888

Nixon, P. (2021, December 14). *Three essential breathing exercises for busy, stressed out moms.* YouAlignedTM. https://youaligned.com/wellness/breath-exercises-stressed-moms

Nocturnal asthma (nighttime asthma). (2022, August 12). WebMD. https://www.webmd.com/asthma/nocturnal-asthma-nighttime-asthma

Nowmedia. (2021, October 20). *How thumb sucking can alter your child's appearance.* Airway and Sleep Group. https://airwayandsleepgroup.com/blog/how-thumb-sucking-can-alter-your-childs-appearance

Oral health and respiratory conditions: The connection revealed. (2023, September 13). Springhill Dentist. https://myspringhilldentist.com/how-are-oral-health-and-respiratory-conditions-connected

Pacheco, D. (2020, October 29). *The best temperature for sleep: Advice and tips.* Sleep Foundation. https://www.sleepfoundation.org/bedroom-environment/best-temperature-for-sleep

Pacheco, D., & Dr. Nilong, V. (2018, October 26). *What is the best way to dress your child for sleep?* Sleep Foundation. https://www.sleepfoundation.org/children-and-sleep/how-to-dress-for-sleep

Parsippany, C. (2024). *Before and after.* DK Ortho. https://dkortho.net/before-and-after

Pediatric obstructive sleep apnea: Symptoms and causes. (2018). Mayo Clinic. https://www.mayoclinic.org/diseases-conditions/pediatric-sleep-apnea/symptoms-causes/syc-20376196

Pelham, V. (2023, Summer 5). *Common breathing problems in kids and how to treat them.* Cedars-Sinai. https://www.cedars-sinai.org/blog/common-breathing-problems-in-kids.html

Phosphorus: How important is this mineral for your teeth and jaws? (2017, November 2). Michael Wasson DMD. https://www.michaelwassondmd.com/phosphorus-how-important-is-this-mineral-for-your-teeth-and-jaws

Price, W. A. (1939). *Nutrition and physical degeneration: A comparison of primitive and modern diets and their effects.* Paul B. Hoeber Inc. Medical Book Department of Harper & Brothers.

Protein and oral health. (n.d.). SmileTown Langley. https://www.smiletownlangley.com/site/blog/2016/07/13/protein-oral-health-teeth-children-nutrition-langley-dentist

Rajini, D. (2023, November 22). *For clearer speech: Effective cheek exercises for kids.* WellnessHub. https://www.mywellnesshub.in/blog/cheek-exercises-speech-language-development

Sendić, G. (2023, October 30). *Respiratory system.* Kenhub. https://www.kenhub.com/en/library/anatomy/the-respiratory-system

Signs of respiratory distress in children. (2014, August 23). Children's Hospital of Philadelphia. https://www.chop.edu/conditions-diseases/signs-respiratory-distress-children

Sinclair, J. (2021, July 12). *How mindful breathing can change your day (and your life).* BetterUp. https://www.betterup.com/blog/mindful-breathing

Snoring in children and toddlers: When to worry. (n.d.). Lurie Children's

Hospital. https://www.luriechildrens.org/en/blog/snoring-in-children-toddlers-when-to-worry

Southern Maine Team. (2023, July 14). *How orthodontics can help with breathing and sleep disorders.* Southern Maine Orthodontics. https://southernmainebraces.com/how-orthodontics-can-help-with-breathing-and-sleep-disorders

Steele, C. (2016, November 21). *No more thumb sucking: Techniques for quitting.* Healthline. https://www.healthline.com/health/parenting/thumb-sucking

Stoustrup, P., Twetman, S., & Varenne, B. (2018). Behavior, oral hygiene, and oral clearance in patients with infantile and juvenile idiopathic scoliosis. *Pediatric Dental Journal, 28(3),* 91–99. https://doi.org/10.1016/j.pdj.2018.07.003

Stressed out? Stop mouth breathing, expert says. (2017, August 2). Fox News. https://www.foxnews.com/health/stressed-out-stop-mouth-breathing-expert-says

Tataryn, M. (2019, February 20). *Tips for optimizing your child's sleep hygiene.* UofM Health Blog. https://healthblog.uofmhealth.org/childrens-health/tips-for-optimizing-your-childs-sleep-hygiene

Teaching kids the importance of posture. (2019, February 11). Swingset Solutions. https://www.swingsetsolutions.net/teaching-kids-the-importance-of-posture/

The benefits of proper breathing. (n.d.). Dardis Communications. *https://www.dardiscommunications.com/2018/11/the-benefits-of-proper-breathing*

The benefits of vitamin D for your teeth and overall oral health. (2022, March 4). Stellalife.com. *https://stellalife.com/blogs/dentamedica-blog/the-benefits-of-vitamin-d-for-your-teeth-and-overall-oral-health*

The growing face of a child (n.d.). Twinkle Dental. *https://twinkledental.com.au/the-growing-face-of-a-child*

The history of orthodontics: From ancient braces to Invisalign. (2021, July 15). Central Coast Orthodontics. *https://centralcoastorthodontics.com.au/the-history-of-orthodontics-from-ancient-braces-to-invisalign*

The importance of early detection: Recognizing signs of respiratory issues. (2023, December 21). Geetanjali Hospital. *https://www.geetanjalihospital.co.in/blogs/view/the-importance-of-early-detection-recognizing-signs-of-respiratory-issues*

The importance of fiber for good oral health. (2016, April 20). EQ Dental. *https://www.eqdental.com/the-importance-of-fiber-for-good-oral-health/*

The importance of good ventilation. (n.d.). EnviroVent Ltd. *https://www.*

envirovent.com/help-and-advice/why-ventilate/indoor-air-quality/the-importance-of-good-ventilation/

The most common posture problems. (2019, November 5). City Chiropractic Clinic. https://city-chiropractic.com/chiropractor-stoke-on-trent/common-posture-problems

The palate. (n.d.). Teach Me Anatomy. https://teachmeanatomy.info/head/other/palate

The stages of sleep. (n.d.). National Sleep Foundation. https://www.sleepfoundation.org/how-sleep-works/stages-of-sleep

Tongue-tie (ankyloglossia). (2021, October 20). Mayo Clinic. https://www.mayoclinic.org/diseases-conditions/tongue-tie/symptoms-causes/syc-20378452

Topiramate: A possible solution for bruxism? (n.d.). The American Academy of Oral Medicine. https://www.aaom.com/index.php?option=com_content&view=article&id=51:topiramate-a-possible-solution-for-bruxism&catid=22:patient-condition-information&Itemid=120

Troxel, W. (2020, February 19). *Does warm milk help you sleep?* Sleep Foundation. https://www.sleepfoundation.org/sleep-hygiene/does-warm-milk-help-you-sleep

Types of malocclusions in children: Everything you need to know. (n.d.). Orthodontic Arts. https://orthodonticarts.com/types-of-malocclusions-in-children-everything-you-need-to-know/

Vitamin C and your teeth. (2017, December 1). TLC Dental. https://www.tlcdental.com.au/blog/2017/12/1/vitamin-c-your-teeth

Wax, J. (2022, March 7). *Nutritional orthodontics: How diet affects your child's smile.* Wax Orthodontics. https://waxorthodontics.com/nutritional-orthodontics-how-diet-affects-your-childs-smile

Sleep stages: The architecture of the night. (2022, September 12). WebMD. https://www.webmd.com/sleep-disorders/guide/sleep-stages

The effects of breathing exercises on blood pressure. (2023, May 2). WebMD. https://www.webmd.com/hypertension-high-blood-pressure/breathing-exercises-lower-blood-pressure

Nocturnal bruxism (teeth grinding): Causes and treatments. (2023, October 11). WebMD. https://www.webmd.com/oral-health/guide/teeth-grinding-bruxism

Weingrow, R. (2022, October 25). *Seven benefits of learning proper posture.* Good Posture. https://www.goodposture.com/blog/7-benefits-of-learning-proper-posture

What are adenoids? (2019, July 3). Nemours KidsHealth. https://kidshealth. org/en/parents/adenoids.html

What are the symptoms of vitamin D deficiency? (2023, September 19). Healthline. https://www.healthline.com/health/food-nutrition/vitamin-d-deficiency-symptoms

What causes snoring in children? (2019, February 20). Verywell Health. https:// www.verywellhealth.com/what-causes-snoring-in-children-4771161

What does a cavity look like? (n.d.). Dental Associates. https://www. dentalassociates.com/blog/what-does-a-cavity-look-like

What is mouth breathing? (2021, October 27). Albee Dental Care. https:// albeedental.com/what-is-mouth-breathing/

What is myofunctional therapy? (2020, May 12). A+ Orthodontics. https:// aplusortho.com/what-is-myofunctional-therapy/

What is myofunctional therapy? (n.d.). Northern Westchester Dental. https:// northernwestchesterdental.com/services/myofunctional-therapy/

What is myofunctional therapy? (n.d.). Northern Westchester Dental. https:// northernwestchesterdental.com/services/myofunctional-therapy/

What is the difference between deep breathing and diaphragmatic breathing? (n.d.). Cornerstone of Hope. https://cornerstoneofhope.org/what-is-the-difference-between-deep-breathing-and-diaphragmatic-breathing/

What's the difference between a mouth breather and a nose breather? (n.d.). The Mayo Clinic Diet. https://diet.mayoclinic.org/diet/expert-answers/ mouth-breather-vs-nose-breather/faq-20425319

What to do about mouth breathing. (2019, February 12). Medical News Today. https://www.medicalnewstoday.com/articles/324496

Why is my child mouth breathing? (2022, February 22). Speech-Language and Learning Center. *https://www.sllcnj.com/why-is-my-child-mouth-breathing/*

Why you need to stop mouth breathing. (n.d.). Sleep Disorders and Therapy. https://sleepdisorders.sleepfoundation.org/other-sleep-disorders/mouth-breathing/

Williams, K. (2019, March 19). *How to help your child sleep comfortably.* UofM Health Blog. https://healthblog.uofmhealth.org/childrens-health/ how-to-help-your-child-sleep-comfortably

Williams, S. (2023, October 30). *The amazing benefits of nasal breathing.* Mouth Breathing. https://www.mouthbreathing.org/breathing-blog/nasal-breathing-benefits

Wolff, L. (2017, June 28). *Ten benefits of correct posture.* Wolf Spinal Care. https://www.wolfspinalcare.com/10-benefits-of-correct-posture

Wood, C. (2021, October 22). *Myofunctional therapy vs traditional orthodontic treatment.* TREC Dental. https://trecdental.com/myofunctional-therapy-vs-traditional-orthodontic-treatment

Young, A. (2021, September 30). *How the tongue affects your dental health.* Arcadia Dental Arts. https://arcadiadentalarts.com/how-the-tongue-affects-your-dental-health/

Made in United States
Troutdale, OR
03/03/2025

29448881R00111